First in Line

How COVID-19 Placed Me on the Frontlines of a Health Care Crisis

SANDRA LINDSAY, RN
WITH JOANNE SKERRETT

A POST HILL PRESS BOOK
ISBN: 979-8-88845-276-9
ISBN (eBook): 979-8-88845-277-6

First in Line:
How COVID-19 Placed Me on the Frontlines of a Health Care Crisis
© 2024 by Sandra Lindsay
All Rights Reserved

Cover design by Jim Villaflores

This book contains advice and information relating to health care. It should be used to supplement rather than replace the advice of your doctor or another trained health professional. You are advised to consult your health professional with regard to matters related to your health, and in particular regarding matters that may require diagnosis or medical attention. All efforts have been made to assure the accuracy of the information in this book as of the date of publication. The publisher and the author disclaim liability for any medical outcomes that may occur as a result of applying the methods suggested in this book.

All people, locations, events, and situations are portrayed to the best of the author's memory. While all of the events described are true, some names and identifying details have been changed to protect the privacy of the people involved.

Post Hill Press
New York • Nashville
posthillpress.com

Published in the United States of America
1 2 3 4 5 6 7 8 9 10

I would like to dedicate this book to the early influencers in my life—my parents Basil Lindsay and Hazel Morgan and my grandparents Norris and Harriet Lindsay. To my son Kadeen Nunes, for teaching me the power of unconditional love, accountability, and responsibility.

CONTENTS

NOTE FROM SANDRA

When I began thinking about this book, I went back and forth on how I would tell my story. Should I focus on my origins and journey from immigrant to COVID-19 vaccine evangelist, or should I grab the opportunity to raise awareness on important social issues that have impacted my life in very real ways? I chose both, and that's what you will read in this book: an immigrant story and a call to action on reducing health disparities in America.

I spent my childhood in Jamaica, where my grandparents and parents raised me and my six siblings, and that shaped me as an individual. I have achieved a lot in America and have earned many academic degrees, beginning with an associate degree in nursing from Borough of Manhattan Community College and, most recently, a doctorate in health sciences. But my associate degree will always be nearest and dearest to my heart. That degree opened the door to my dream of being a nurse and enabled me to have this thirty-year nursing career. Health care has always been my passion and calling, first as a kid caring for my sick grandmother and now as an executive in a top hospital system.

I truly hope this book reflects my desire to see that the disadvantaged experience the benefits of healthy living and equitable health care as much as it reflects my journey as an immigrant, struggling for decades with minimum-wage jobs and part-time school and climbing from the poverty line to a position of relative wealth. While I hope that part of my story will inspire others to make their own version of the American dream come true, that would not be the full story.

When I became an American citizen, it was such a proud day because as much as I love Jamaica, I believe I was not giving up that part of myself but gaining another part of myself. I believe this country affords most people the opportunity to do great things. But for some, the barriers to achieving great things, sometimes even normal things, like finding healthy food or a doctor who listens to their concerns, can be very high.

While living in the Bronx in the late '80s and '90s, I experienced the frustrations and indignity of being poor. But even with all the success I have achieved, I still face obstacles; I still experience discrimination as a woman of color. I do not see myself as a victim in the least, but I am a realist. I overcame, but it wasn't easy. My dream is to see equitable treatment for the disadvantaged in society without the hefty emotional cost or the unnecessary struggle.

This is a story about my life: my family, my early years in Jamaica, my life in America for the last forty years or so, the COVID-19 pandemic as I experienced it, and how my passions and priorities changed after I became the first person in North America to take the COVID-19 vaccine. This is also a story about health disparities and health-care problems faced by disadvantaged communities, including chronic disease, mental illness, and maternal and infant mortality.

At the end of this book, I hope to have raised awareness of the impact of health-care disparities on regular people and how we can be better advocates for ourselves and live healthier, happier lives. That is my goal in sharing my story. I hope you will be inspired by it, not just as another professional success story but as a call to action to address the problem of health-care inequity in our society.

Part I

THE BIG PICTURE

CHAPTER 1

Medal Ceremony

I woke up in a hotel room near the White House on July 7, 2022, in a state of nervousness. In a matter of hours, I would be awarded the Presidential Medal of Freedom along with sixteen other decorated and accomplished Americans. I re-rehearsed the protocols I had received in an email with the address "whitehouse.gov" just a week ago. As I dressed, I checked everything twice: makeup carefully done in the wee hours of the morning by my niece Ashanti, a young brilliant special education teacher, who had traveled from Albany with my sister and her four other siblings to cheer me on and babysit her siblings Amari, Amore, Amir, and baby Asher while my sister attended the ceremony, my suit buttons, the middle part in my hair; I made sure nothing was stuck between my teeth. So many people were rooting for me, supporting me, cheering me on from back home.

My mother Hazel, sister Flavia, friend Pauline, Matt Libassi, Northwell's public relations manager who was with me since the first shot, and Her Excellency Audrey Marks, ambassador of Jamaica to the US were with me, and I certainly didn't want to embarrass them on national TV. Sadly, my son Kadeem had to travel back to New York for an emergency and could not attend the ceremony in person and my auntie Marie tested positive for COVID the day before the ceremony and had to tearfully watch on TV. She was so proud of me, but she was really looking forward to getting a glimpse, a handshake, or perhaps a selfie with Denzel Washington, her favorite actor. Most of all, I couldn't disappoint the memory of my grandparents who raised me. These people were my cloud of witnesses who steadied me as I put away my doubts and prepared to go into the ceremony.

Sixteen hundred Pennsylvania Avenue is a long way from where I grew up with six siblings in my grandparents' house in Jamaica. Maybe I was right to allow myself a moment of panic and to ask myself: What was I doing here, just a few feet away from the leader of the free world, about to receive one of the most venerated civilian honors? It wasn't the first time I would be on a stage with President Joe Biden. In 2021, I was awarded the US Citizenship and Immigration Services Outstanding Americans by Choice award at the White House soon after I became the first person in the United States to receive the Pfizer COVID-19 vaccine, but this honor felt different. I felt proud, humbled, excited, nervous, and pensive all at once.

I have been a registered nurse since 1994 when I joined Northwell Health's Lenox Hill Hospital in the oncology department. It was my dream job at the time, achieved after years of struggle. When I moved to the United States in 1986 at age eighteen, I had no idea what the future held for me and my dreams. I was the girl studying on the subway, shuttling between odd jobs while taking classes at Borough of Manhattan Community College. Studying, working, studying, working. I did not dream of meeting the president of the United States. I dreamed of having a fulfilling career that would allow me to lead a comfortable life, own a home, and take a few nice vacations. Obviously, I got exceedingly more than I wished.

The medal ceremony is both solemn and celebratory. A military band played "All Hail the Chief" as the president entered the room, and we—the medal recipients seated on the stage and the full room of press and family members—stood to applaud him. Cindy McCain, the wife of the late US Senator John McCain, sat to my left. It felt like I was in a dream.

As a child growing up in Jamaica, my heroes were my grandparents, who instilled in me the importance of good character, diligence, courage, and confidence. They were ordinary people who encouraged me to believe I could do extraordinary things. So, here I was on that humid July day, starstruck amid these internationally known figures. There was Fred Gray, a lawyer and politician who represented Rosa Parks, the NAACP, and Martin Luther King Jr. over the course of his career. Gabrielle Giffords, the former congresswoman from Arizona, was honored for her political career and founding of a nonprofit that works for gun violence prevention. I was more than impressed to meet accomplished soccer player Megan Rapinoe and gymnast Simone Biles, whose advocacy for mental health inspires me as much as her gravity-defying athletic achievements. And did I mention that one of my favorite actors, Denzel Washington, was among the honorees?

Yes, I had come quite a long way. The photographers and reporters in the room, the uniformed servicemen and women stationed at the edges, and the array of American flags reminded me of that fact. There was greatness all around me, an ordinary person, a naturalized American who loves her adopted country and believes strongly in its ideals.

When I agreed to take the COVID-19 vaccine in December 2020, I did not see myself as a hero. I, like most ordinary people, simply wanted the pandemic to end. I simply did what many Americans do when faced with the unknown: I researched and informed myself of the risks, spoke with my loved ones and health-care providers, and then took action. My family was supportive. My brother was even ecstatic, and my son was doubtful at first but proud of me for putting myself on the front line.

REMEMBERING THE FALLEN

As the medal ceremony went on, I allowed myself to relax and appreciate the honorees and their stories. When it was my turn to step forward, I made sure to smile—for my loved ones who were in the room or cheering me on from afar. I only partly heard what the announcer read about me, but I did catch the part when he called me a "ray of light" and said that I "represented the best of America." I so wished my grandparents could have been alive to witness that moment.

Yet, as proud as I was at that moment at the White House, I could not help but think of the nearly seven million people worldwide who had lost their lives because of the COVID-19 virus. In March 2020, I saw firsthand the devastation of the pandemic as I led a team of nurses at Northwell Health, which was, for a time, the nation's epicenter of the pandemic. So many friends, mothers, fathers, siblings, and coworkers were lost before vaccines became available. Our fallen heroes and their grieving loved ones were on my mind as President Biden placed the medal around my neck. I was grateful for sure, and I was also determined to never forget each of those lives and to continue to advocate for a better, more equitable health-care system.

Today, many people feel that COVID-19 is no longer an acute threat, even though it still lurks among us. Life has mostly returned to normal around the world, and I, like most people, shudder when I recall the uncertainty and darkness of the spring of 2020. Many of our friends and neighbors continue to suffer from the effects of long COVID-19, families are still mourning empty seats at dinner tables, and political debates around vaccines and the virus itself threaten to divide our communities. The pandemic revealed so many of our weaknesses, and it would be a shame if we rushed to move past it without attempting to heal our many ailments as a society.

WHY I AM WRITING THIS BOOK

In a statement about the medal ceremony, President Biden said America can be defined by one word—"possibilities"—adding that the honorees "demonstrate the power of possibilities and embody the soul of the nation—hard work, perseverance, and faith." I wholeheartedly agree with President Biden regarding the Medal of Freedom recipients. But I can also attest to the many unsung citizens I have met in my nearly three decades in health care who pursue their goals and dreams in the face of illness, poverty, and a health-care system that seems stacked against them. Even before the devastation of COVID-19, I had long felt a burden for those struggling with ill health and inadequate access to health care, many of them poor and people of color. These hardworking Americans want to enjoy the best of what this country has to offer but are sometimes held back by inequities in our health-care system. Their daily struggles and perseverance inspired me to write this book to encourage us all to care and advocate for the vulnerable in our communities.

Despite the fact that the United States has the world's foremost health-care institutions, Americans who live in lower-income areas, many of them people of color, tend to suffer worse health outcomes than their white counterparts and face insurmountable barriers to accessing proper health care. Minority patients' outcomes can be attributed to "lower quality and intensity of healthcare and diagnostic services across a wide range of procedures and disease areas,"[1] according to researchers. These disparities in care and access manifest themselves in higher infant mortality rates, higher prevalence of chronic diseases such as diabetes, cardiovascular illnesses, cancers, and a higher likelihood of death from these diseases for Black people compared to Whites.[2]

This is not a problem that can be solved simply by eating right, exercising, and pulling oneself up by the bootstraps. Health-care inequities also arise in the way marginalized people perceive mistreatment in their encounters with the health-care system. One of the leading researchers of the impact of social inequality on health has written that social disadvantage on its own can lead to poorer health outcomes for individuals.

---

[1]   Brian D. Smedley, Adrienne Y. Stith, and Alan R. Nelson, editors, "Unequal Treatment: Confronting Racial and Ethnic Disparities in Health Care," National Library of Medicine, National Academies Press, Washington, DC, 2003, p. 70, https://pubmed. ncbi.nlm.nih.gov/25032386/.

[2]   "Key Facts on Health and Health Care by Race and Ethnicity," KFF, January 26, 2022, https:// www.kff.org/racial-equity-and-health-policy/press-release/key-facts-on-health-and-health-care-by-race-and-ethnicity/.

The result of unequal distribution of life chances is that health is unequally distributed. If you are born in the most fortunate circumstances you can expect to have your healthy life extended by nineteen years or more, compared with being born into disadvantage. Being at the wrong end of equality is disempowering. It deprives people of control over their lives. Their health is damaged as a result. And the effect is graded—the greater the disadvantage the worse the health.

–Professor Sir Michael Marmot, author of
The Health Gap: The Challenge of an Unequal World (Bloomsbury: 2015)

Indeed, progress has been made on several fronts, but much remains to be done. For example, a well-known study that examined the black-white mortality gap between 1960 and 2000 found that a startling 83,570 deaths (using 2000 data) could be prevented in the US each year if the black-white mortality gap was eliminated.[3] The black-white life expectancy gap has narrowed by nearly 50 percent in the last three decades from seven years to 3.6 years,[4] meaning more Black people are living longer. But health disparities persist in our nation, and COVID-19 sadly robbed us of many of the gains made over the last few decades. Today, the entire nation faces health challenges. Here are some chilling statistics that should concern all of us:

- **Life expectancy is declining:** According to the Centers for Disease Control and Prevention, life expectancy at birth in the United States declined nearly a year from 2020 to 2021. That

---

[3] David Satcher, et al., "What If We Were Equal? A Comparison of the Black-White Mortality Gap in 1960 and 2000," *Health Affairs (Project Hope)*, vol. 24, no. 2 (March-April 2005): 459–64, https://doi.org/10.1377/hlthaff.24.2.459.

[4] B. Rose Huber, "Life Expectancy Gap Between Black and White Americans Closes Nearly 50% in 30 Years," Princeton School of Public and International Affairs, September 28, 2021, https://spia.princeton.edu/news/life-expectancy-gap-between-black-and-white-americans-closes-nearly-50-30-years.

decline—77.0 to 76.1 years—took US life expectancy at birth to its lowest level since 1996. The 0.9-year drop in life expectancy in 2021, along with a 1.8-year drop in 2020, was the biggest two-year decline in life expectancy since 1921–1923.[5]

- **Despite gains, millions are still uninsured:** The Affordable Care Act has increased the number of Americans who have insurance, but in certain states that have not expanded Medicaid eligibility under the act, the number of insured people continues to lag. According to the US Census, out of the thirty-six states and the District of Columbia that have expanded Medicaid eligibility on or before January 1, 2021, the uninsured rate was 6.6 percent, but that rate was 12 percent or more in states that had not expanded Medicaid eligibility under the Affordable Care Act.[6]

THE POWER OF POSSIBILITIES

In the last few years, people around the globe have shared with me their COVID-19 experiences, chronic health struggles, and challenges with hospitals, insurers, and even health-care professionals. I've also spent countless hours with dedicated nurses like me who are facing burnout, brought to the point of breaking from overwork and hostility from an increasingly polarized public. Our health-care system is in desperate need of healing.

There is so much to be done. We can do more to close the gaps in health equity, improve the health outcomes for our vulnerable citizens, and place more value on our health-care professionals. As President Biden said, America is a nation of possibilities, and our spirit of possibility should be quickened when we see our vulnerable neighbors suffering.

---

5   "Life Expectancy in the U.S. Dropped for the Second Year in a Row in 2021," Centers for Disease Control and Prevention, August 31, 2022, https://www.cdc.gov/nchs/pressroom/nchs_press_releases/2022/20220831.htm.

6   "Uninsured Rate Declined in 28 States 2019-2021," US Census Bureau, September 15, 2022, https://www.census.gov/library/stories/2022/09/uninsured-rate-declined-in-28-states.html.

I can no longer sit by idly and enjoy the good life now that I'm aware of the problems my communities face. Neither can you. Whether as an advocate for our family and friends or in spreading awareness as health-care providers, we can all play a part.

As you read this book and get to know more about my life, my experiences in the health-care industry, and the causes that I am passionate about, I hope we together develop an understanding of the scope and impact of health disparities in our nation and how ordinary people like us can be part of the solution by simply caring more for our vulnerable friends and neighbors.

I got vaccinated because I have always believed in leading by example. As I witnessed from the front line the mass devastation of COVID-19, taking the vaccine was an obvious choice. Taking action was what I learned from my grandmother, my mother, my father, a compassionate public servant, and my mentors, and I hope this book will inspire you to act as well.

CHAPTER 2

Seven Men in Chronic Distress

I am often asked: What was the absolute worst day of the COVID-19 crisis for you as a health-care professional? The answer is there wasn't one particular day. When I think back to spring 2020, my mind knits together separate incidents and scenes that span the two-year crisis: colleagues' faces and bodies shrouded in PPE, weeping families staring through iPad screens at dying loved ones, terrified voices announcing rapid response after rapid response after rapid response over the hospital PA system, and emotions, lots of emotions. The difficult things my team and I experienced are not easily put into words. And I certainly do not want to make a spectacle out of the suffering of the patients who came to our critical care units. So, as I relate these stories, my goal will always be to motivate others to act while doing my best to respect and honor the very real people that we lost and their grieving loved ones.

In March of early 2020, when the first wave of COVID-19 hit, I was the director of the critical care division at Northwell Health's Long Island Jewish Medical Center (LIJMC), a job I considered a dream role when I started in March 2016. Before COVID-19, there were five units under my responsibility and four nurse managers who reported to me directly. Each nurse manager had three to four assistant nurse managers who reported directly to them but fell under my purview in addition to the nurse managers and assistant nurse managers. My responsibilities spanned all these managers and their staff over the five units, including patient care associates, unit receptionists, and support staff who cared for the patients brought in from the emergency department and other parts of the hospital, other hospitals within and outside of Northwell, and inpatient units within LIJMC.

On March 11, 2020, the World Health Organization (WHO) declared the COVID-19 outbreak a global pandemic, but in the days before that, the rapidly increasing volume of patients told us as such. Northwell, as an integrated Health System of more than twenty hospitals, was doing everything possible to find patient beds and equipment and keep up with staffing and patient care needs. The excellent leadership of the Northwell health network had long prepared for a crisis like COVID-19, even applying lessons from the aftermath of the attacks on the World Trade Center in New York City on September 11, 2001. Through every stage of the COVID-19 emergency, Northwell's Incident Command agilely coordinated a multifaceted response to the outbreak among the several hospitals in the Northwell network, but that executive strategy was way above me and my pay grade.

On the ground level where my staff and I operated, every day came another challenge, another bleak horizon that we had to plow through. The steady stream of patients tested the nursing staff to the breaking point, and for weeks, we were exhausted, overwhelmed, operating on little sleep, and running on pure adrenaline. Many times, I had to break the bad news to the nurse managers that we needed more overtime shifts covered or that we were opening up a new ICU unit and might have to work very late. Meanwhile, patients kept coming to us sicker and sicker.

I was laser-focused on running the division efficiently and making sure the team could do their work with as few hiccups as possible in this chaotic environment. It might sound strange, but the patients were sort of abstract figures to me those first couple of weeks in March. Maybe it's because I hadn't yet fully appreciated the scale of what was coming. Truthfully, I viewed COVID-19 as something that would go away within a couple of weeks or a month. I thought all we had to do was to get through the next few weeks, and this emergency would blow over— like the H1N1 or Zika virus. Finding more beds, staffing a twelve-hour shift, ensuring that the staff had all the tools and equipment to do their job safely—those things were somewhat in my control and thus easier to focus on. I was so busy I could not slow down enough to think about the people in the beds we were working so hard to save.

One morning, that changed. I was on rounds with our team on yet another bad day when uncertainty and urgency began and ended every shift. Although we were handling it with all the professionalism we could muster, morning rounds were tough and disheartening. Many patients we had seen the day before would be gone; they had not lived through the night.

That particular morning, I was forced to slow down. There, in one of the ICUs I managed, I counted seven middle-aged Black men fighting for their lives right in front of me. The room was dimly lit and still, so still, except for the sound of the machinery, the hiss of oxygen being fed to their lungs. They wore hospital gowns, and each one was on a ventilator. The staff had lain them either supine or prone on their beds to facilitate better air exchange.

The sight of these men stopped me in my tracks. Those seven men lying helpless, silent, and unable to breathe on their own grabbed me deep inside. My God, I thought. More and more people of color were coming into the ICU, I realized. This was no longer a virus that was claiming the lives of people in China or elderly Italians thousands of miles away. These people dying by the tens daily looked like my neighbors, like my family members, like me. What was happening? Was this going to be it for our community? Were we all going to be cut down by this virus?

Troubled and distracted, I followed the team through the motions of rounds and then tried to get into my tasks for the day. I couldn't shake the image of those seven men, however, as I began to pay closer attention to the types of patients in the ICU, on ventilators, waiting for a bed. Those seven men—silent, sedated, and isolated—were regular guys, men I would have seen when I lived in the Bronx as a new immigrant to the US in 1986. They were men I could have worked with or for over my long career as a nurse. They probably sat next to me on planes or on the subway. They were men just like my brother, my father, my son.

I went back later to take a closer look at their charts, as I would for other patients in the following weeks. The common thread in those charts? Chronic conditions like diabetes, heart disease, and hypertension. Within that first week in March and over the ensuing weeks, many more patients fitting that profile would come to the ICU.[7] These patients were not only lower-income folks. They worked in public-facing jobs, were essential workers, took public transportation, were international travelers, and had pre-existing medical conditions. In those early days, many patients did not make it out of the ICU, and it did not take long before those seven men passed away as well.

I often think about those seven men and the lives they lived, the children they raised, the parents who raised them, their coworkers, neighbors, girlfriends, partners, or wives. I am sure they are missed by their loved ones to this day. Those seven men are among many others we lost that I will never forget.

Those bodies on stretchers being ferried away to the morgue or to refrigerated trucks on the loading dock on the LIJMC campus were no longer just bodies. They were real people who were among the first to lose their lives in the pandemic that was turning the world upside down.

LOCKED DOWN IN FEAR

During March 2020, people were terrified, and rightly so. A virus was claiming lives all over the world, and there was no cure and few ways to protect oneself from it. Since February, we had been glued to our phones

---

[7] While many of our sickest patients already had serious health issues, I am not sharing this incident to make correlations between COVID-19 and chronic disease.

or TVs constantly, desperate for good news, brought low by the ticking counters marking the number of infected, the number of dead, and the deadly projections for next week, next month.

We were forced to stay indoors, only allowed in the grocery store at certain hours, and prohibited from attending school, church, or the gym. There was nothing normal about that time, and our society will never be the same because of it. We were isolated from all the normal things that we previously took for granted: work and school relationships with people different from us, neighborly chats, choir practice, book clubs, and dining out. All the things that brought us together as human beings came to a screeching halt.

Our way of life was threatened, up in the air, and we did not know when things would return to normal. The authorities certainly didn't seem to know. The two-week shutdown turned into four weeks, then months until we could "flatten the curve." The message on masking changed every other week, it seemed. Politics began to compete with and overrun the public health discussion. There was so much fear, sadness, and confusion during that time. It's a wonder we kept our sanity.

When news of a possible vaccine began to circulate in the news, I was excited, and so were many of my colleagues. Trust me, I had no plans or desire to become a national advocate for vaccination. All I knew was I wanted the deaths to stop; I wanted work to be normal again; I wanted to be able to see my mom, my son, and grandson regularly; I wanted to drop the mask, and I wanted COVID-19 to disappear for good, never to be heard from again! Those were my main motivations. Too many people were still suffering, and our lives were still far from normal. We needed a solution, and I felt fortunate to be a part of it.

A MAJOR THREAT TO HEALTH

Vaccine hesitancy was named one of the top ten threats to global health in 2019 by the WHO, but almost a decade before, in 2010, global health officials finally acknowledged the reality of public mistrust in vaccines in the wake of the H1N1 virus.[8] Vaccine hesitancy persisted, the WHO found, because of complacency, inconvenience in accessing vaccines, and lack of confidence in medicine and the health-care industry. Before the Bill Gates microchip and other far-fetched conspiracies cluttered our social media feeds, vaccine hesitancy was imperiling the health of many across the globe. Fast-forward to the present, and vaccine hesitancy has become even more widespread.

But the fact is, vaccines do work. Vaccination is one of the most cost-effective ways of avoiding disease and prevents two to three million deaths a year worldwide. A further 1.5 million deaths could be avoided if global coverage of vaccinations improved, according to the WHO.[9]

There was a tremendous amount of vaccine advocacy work done by government, nonprofit, and private-sector organizations during the COVID-19 pandemic. I'm sure you remember seeing TV spots from the Ad Council and other organizations urging you to get vaccinated. Some efforts were more effective than others, but they all made an impact, at least from the data. The CDC's National Immunization Survey of people eighteen years or older who received at least one dose of the COVID-19 vaccine showed that 89 percent of African Americans had received the vaccine, a higher percentage than that of Whites (data collected from April 2021 to March 2023).[10] That number is a striking achievement, I believe, particularly considering the weight of the history of medical exploitation in our community and the toxic politicization and controversy around the COVID-19 vaccine. Our community should truly be proud. I am only hopeful that we will continue to be open to vaccines in the future.

[8]   Heidi J. Larson, Emmanuela Gakidou, and Christopher J.L. Murray, "The Vaccine-Hesitant Moment," *New England Journal of Medicine*, 387 (July 7, 2022): 58–65, https://www.nejm.org/doi/full/10.1056/nejmra2106441.

[9]   "Ten Threats to Global Health in 2019," World Health Organization, https://www.who.int/news-room/spotlight/ten-threats-to-global-health-in-2019.

[10]   "Trends in Demographic Characteristics of People Receiving COVID-19 Vaccinations in the United States," Centers for Disease Control and Prevention, https://covid.cdc.gov/covid-data-tracker/#vaccination-demographics-trends.

However, there are still millions of people who have not taken the COVID-19 vaccine, including the elderly and people with comorbidities who do not feel compelled to have their booster shots. CDC data from a study covering twenty-five jurisdictions over the last three months of 2021 showed that the death rate was fifty-three times higher among the unvaccinated than for people who had received booster shots.[11] Unfortunately, as the virus slowly faded from the headlines, apathy and complacency seemed to have taken hold, and many continue to hold on to their convictions that the vaccine is dangerous, ineffective, or somehow sinister. Who would have thought that a vaccine could cause so much controversy and division in our families and communities?

---

[11]   Aaron Blake, "Yes, It's Still a Pandemic of the Unvaccinated — Arguably Even More So Now," *Washington Post*, February 3, 2022, https://www.washingtonpost.com/politics/2022/02/03/yes-its-still-pandemic-unvaccinated-arguably-even-more-so-now/.

CHAPTER 3

My Anti-Vax Friends

I have always tried to be an optimist. During the worst of the pandemic, when the hospital units were overfilled with sick patients, and ambulances were screeching outside, bringing in even more, I tried to keep my team motivated, reminding them that we were our patients' last hope even though we ourselves were terrified of being infected. I am so proud of these nurses and staff members who did not place their fears ahead of their purpose.

I was one of several Northwell staffers who was willing in December 2020 to step forward to take the COVID-19 vaccine—not because I was ignorant of the brutal and complex history of medical exploitation or the various theories on the dangers of vaccines generally.[12] I believed in my heart that it was the right thing to do, and I was well aware that not everyone shared my belief.

---

[12] In a later chapter, I will discuss enslaved and other marginalized people whose bodies were used, without their informed consent, to develop many of the medical advances we have today. I will also discuss the enslaved Africans on Caribbean plantations who shared their West African medical practices and knowledge with European plantation doctors.

SCARY, UNCERTAIN TIMES CAN BREED MISTRUST

The COVID-19 pandemic exposed weaknesses in our government, public health system, and media. With mixed messaging on mask-wearing, botched distribution of government-issued test kits, a lack of clarity on opening/closing schools and businesses, the spread of misinformation on social media and traditional media, and uneven access to the vaccines, it's no wonder that we were targeting and thinking the worst of one another.

Did you ever feel that people were judging you simply because you asked questions about the COVID-19 vaccines? Did you ever gossip about your coworker or neighbor who didn't sign up to get vaccinated within the first week of vaccine availability in your town? Are you still not on speaking terms with your friend from high school who posted those conspiracy theories on Facebook? Well, you're not alone. Although, you should be! We need to get past all this polarization and not let these issues divide us. As strongly as I advocate for vaccines, I do not believe that these disagreements are worth sacrificing our close relationships.

STILL MAD AS HELL

Today, some friends who had refused to take the vaccine remain defiant, others feel vindicated because many of their vaccinated friends ultimately were infected with the virus. Many remain defensive and, to this day, send me websites with obscure studies from even more obscure scientists. My goal in these conversations and interactions has never been to prove that I am right but to always listen and lead with love. As much as I continue to believe that the COVID-19 vaccines helped save millions of lives, I still want to respect the people who did not trust the vaccines. I believe, to this day, that listening to people and asking respectful questions can do a lot to change minds or at least get my friends to begin to see a different point of view.

Trust me: anger and mockery will not work. Nor will shaming and guilt-tripping. I had to take a firm line sometimes, though. Look, I said to some friends, I took so many vaccines as a kid growing up in Jamaica, not knowing what they were and what they would do. We're facing a killer here; I don't have time to argue conspiracy theories when hundreds of thousands of people are dying!

I counted out winning over the many people who've long been suspicious of vaccines for various reasons, some they felt were in their best health interests. Those people are just harder to convince, have strongly held beliefs, and tend to be immersed in the literature supporting their point of view. For instance, some people were concerned about mercury poisoning in vaccines generally and came out strongly against the COVID-19 vaccines as a result. Others wanted to maintain a completely natural lifestyle—no chemicals of any kind would be allowed in their bodies.

The people who were misinformed and held wrong beliefs about the COVID-19 vaccines stood a better chance of being persuaded by the facts. For me, misinformation was an opportunity for conversation. I wasn't impatient and angry with them. They seemed to me a lot like difficult patients I'd encountered throughout my career. I lost two family members to COVID-19 early in the pandemic and watched hundreds of sick patients die for over a year so of course I wanted everyone to take the vaccine. But my decades of experience in health care told me that this would not be a slam dunk argument to win over everyone, especially in the polarized times we were living in.

When I hear the reasons of my vaccine-hesitant friends, I don't always hear stubbornness or craziness. I hear reasonable concerns, and I sympathize with their cautiousness and their intelligent questions. Many of us know colleagues who lost their jobs because of refusing to accept vaccination; some lost relationships and were mocked and harassed. These were strongly held beliefs that those of us who disagreed with them should not lightly set aside.

IN THEIR OWN WORDS

Here is the testimony of a young Black woman in her twenties who lost job opportunities because she refused to take the vaccine. I asked her to write down the reasons why, and these are her own words:

- It did not take long for a new vaccine to be made. The timing was suspicious. There was not enough testing, evaluation, or proof that it works to prevent, cure, or get rid of the disease. Everything was put together so fast, and it was being required for everyone to take it.
- Piggybacking off the first point, no one knows the effects of the vaccine in the long run. It could be super detrimental. No one knows the long-term effects.
- They were offering gifts and money to the first few people to take it. That seemed pretty sketchy because I personally don't recall getting offered gifts for taking other vaccines. This vaccine has been pushed so heavily and abruptly down everyone's throat.
- America's history of using Black people as test subjects for their studies. Example: Tuskegee Study and another article detailing what happened in Africa with the injecting of diseases without their consent or knowledge.
- People have gotten the vaccine and still got COVID-19. That in itself swayed me away from getting the vaccine.
- I don't know how my body would react to that new vaccine in my body and whether I would experience any side effects.

This young woman was not belligerent or angry; she seemed very calm the few times we talked. She admitted that she got most of her information about the COVID-19 vaccine from online articles and sources that were not mainstream media like CBS or FOX News or CNN. She watched YouTube and TikTok videos shared by her friends from high school and college and people she knew from gaming websites. These videos and articles from her friends pushed theories that the COVID-19 vaccines were not tested adequately, were unsafe, could negatively affect human DNA, and that the side effects were unknown.

She admitted that she trusted these sources more than she did government officials and the traditional media. "I feel that videos on TikTok are not censored by the government. I think they (the government) would not tell us the truth about what was really going on with COVID-19 and how the vaccine came about."

Asked whether her view was influenced by politics she said no. "I'm not a right-wing person. I consider myself a liberal on most issues, but I just think the government was not being upfront with the country, so I didn't feel confident taking the vaccine."

What about other people and their fears of being infected, I said. Weren't you concerned about them? "I wore masks all the time and mostly stayed indoors," she said. "I also did weekly testing, so I never felt bad about what people were saying about unvaccinated people." She noted that she is still careful and wears a mask on the subway and in other public places, even in 2023. Asked how she felt about people who were very pro-vaccine and who came out strongly against people who refused to take the vaccine, she shrugged. "Everyone is entitled to their opinion. I didn't take it (the name calling) as a personal attack."

NO JUDGMENT, JUST CONVERSATION

Does this sound like an unreasonable person to you? A murderer? Not to me. I did my best to explain to her that the vaccine technologies used in the Moderna and Pfizer-BioNTech COVID-19 vaccines have been in development since the early 2000s, with the research going back many decades.[13] Not only that, the unprecedented level of coordination of resources—from the government, private industry, manufacturing, research, and health care—that went into developing and delivering the vaccines is something that has never been seen. But she was not convinced.

I couldn't understand why people were ripping each other to shreds over whether or not they took the vaccine. It was clear that what should have been a public health issue had been taken over by a toxic political moment. Now that we have had some distance from 2020 and all

---

[13] "Decades in the Making: mRNA COVID-19 Vaccines," National Institutes of Health, https://covid19.nih.gov/nih-strategic-response-covid-19/decades-making-mrna-covid-19-vaccines.

its trauma, drama, and confusion, maybe we can think about having a better conversation about vaccination in our families, communities, workplaces, and institutions and mend some of the relationships that were broken or cracked because of these petty arguments.

One of the saddest realizations for me throughout this saga was just the sheer number of young and marginalized people who were falling prey to misinformation on social media about the vaccine. The Internet offered so many opportunities for people to organize themselves around politics, religion, hobbies, and other affinities while we were quarantined, but there was a dark side to that as well.

I know of very religious people in my community who said that the vaccine represented an apocalyptic sign from the book of Revelation in the Bible. Some thought it would be against their faith to take the vaccine. They did not like to be reminded that they had taken vaccines for measles, mumps, and other common infections without raising these religious convictions. Even some young celebrities got into the act of spreading misinformation, warning that the vaccine would cause infertility or autism. It was shocking (and amusing) to me that sensible-seeming people were firmly confident that the vaccine had negative effects, although it was untested and unproven in every other way. I don't mean to make fun of people, but it was a very frustrating and scary time.

THE OTHER SIDE OF THE DEBATE

A veteran nurse friend who works with the elderly at a long-term health facility is staunchly pro-vaccine and believes that all health-care workers should be vaccinated without exception. It's hard enough seeing elderly people living out their last years struggling with sickness, she said. COVID-19 added a new dimension of risk and suffering for those patients and made her job even more challenging.

Like me, she was relieved when the COVID-19 vaccines were finally announced and available. In her professional context, she was ecstatic that the elderly and first responders were given first priority. "I had no hesitation," she said about taking the vaccine herself. She thinks that disagreements over the vaccine have broken up families and caused rifts in communities that may never be repaired. I hope she is wrong. Here are some of her perspectives.

- Most of our (nursing) staff was vaccinated once they became available.
- We were tested every day before the shift. So, you would know within fifteen minutes before your shift if you had it or not. There were resistant groups, both staff and patients. People would just decide, okay, I'm not gonna get vaccinated.
- It was sad because when some of our patients were really sick with the virus, that's when they wanted the vaccine, and they would ask us to give it to them. But we couldn't do anything for them at that point.
- Personally, I didn't want to be near people who were not vaccinated. Too many members of my family never got the vaccine, and to this day, I wear a mask when I'm near them. I refused to share a hotel room with a family member during our family reunion because she never got the vaccine. I am still being careful. At the family reunion, I didn't want anyone kissing or hugging me. I still don't shake hands. I went on a job interview once, and I told them right off the bat that I don't shake hands, and they were fine with that. I think they understood.
- My partner and I were having problems before the pandemic started, but COVID-19 made things worse. In some ways, I would say COVID-19 sped up our divorce. My partner is definitely anti-vax and was reading all kinds of stuff online and sharing anti-vax stuff on Facebook. We hardly saw each other because I was working and didn't want to expose them to the virus. We stayed on separate floors of the house for most of the year.

MEDIA AND MESSAGING

It is too late to ban the Internet, I think, or else that would be one of my policy proposals, and while social media can and has been used to spread misinformation regarding vaccines, those same digital networks are providing data and information to researchers who study how to decrease mistrust in vaccines and increase levels of trust in the public. Despite the controversies tied to the pandemic, studies have found that doctors and nurses still retain a high level of trust[14] among the public, so it is up to us as health-care providers to respect our friends and families when they voice their concerns about vaccinations and to explain to them the facts with respect.

My passion continues to be educating the public about the power of vaccines to save lives. I want to increase the trust and communication with friends, family, and our communities, and that will only come by listening and respecting one another.

LEARNING FROM MISTAKES

One thing that helped me with explaining to friends and family why they should take the vaccine was providing answers to their questions and admitting when I didn't know the answer. I tried to point them to the experts who could answer their specific questions, whether in my workplace or from my academic life. As a medical professional, that was easier for me, and you may have to be more creative.

In 2021, when I began to do public events to encourage people to get vaccinated, I was always realistic about people and human nature in general. That realism probably comes from nearly three decades in nursing and dealing with patients from all levels of society. I knew it would be an uphill battle to get us, meaning the United States, to a 75 percent vaccination rate, which was the goal at the time. The rhetoric and

---

[14] Heidi J. Larson, Emmanuela Gakidou, and Christopher J.L. Murray, "The Vaccine-Hesitant Moment," *New England Journal of Medicine*, 387 (July 7, 2022): 58–65, https://www.nejm.org/doi/full/10.1056/nejmra2106441.

controversy were raw, but I believed in the message that we could stop the spread of COVID-19 and its deadly effects. As I explained to several media outlets, my strategy was first to lead with love. I never wanted anyone to feel ashamed for being hesitant to take the vaccine. I believed that getting into the relationship and having a conversation—or several—could move hesitant people closer to at least considering the vaccine.

Even today, I continue to encourage people to take the vaccine. I remind them that we are back to our busy, connected, fun lives largely because of the vaccines. And even though we are back to "normal," people are still being infected with and dying from COVID-19. So, yes, get your booster.

I have not stopped beating the drum for vaccination, and I never will. When I came to America in 1986 as an eighteen-year-old, I simply wanted to be a nurse to care for hurting people and to champion them when they regained their health. When I think back on the barriers I faced—and overcame—I am energized about the future and what is possible, whether it's convincing more people to consider vaccination or persuading public officials to act on health-care disparities and health inequities in our country.

Part II

COMING TO AMERICA

CHAPTER 4

Coming to America

Just as I had dreamed, I arrived to a white Christmas in New York City in December 1986, leaving behind sunny Jamaica and my very sheltered life. For months, I had imagined what the snow would look like and how it would feel on my skin, and I wondered whether New York would be like every Hollywood movie I'd seen. Would I hear Frank Sinatra crooning, New York, New York! in the background? Would I stare open-mouthed at the glass, chrome, and steel skyscrapers over the gray Hudson River? And would I feel awed by the aura of money, power, and endless opportunity cloaking it all? Well, it wasn't like that—not even close. My flight landed late at night; I was exhausted, freezing, and already homesick. My older sister and cousin picked me up from JFK in my cousin's minivan, shuttled me off to my sister's apartment in the Bronx, and I quickly fell asleep, anxiously awaiting morning to see what the place really looked like.

I woke not to virgin snowflakes and whimsically decorated store windows of Thirty-Fourth Street but to a bustling, noisy section off Fordham Road in the Bronx. Buses hissed and groaned as they passed every few minutes. Pedestrians in puffy jackets carrying bags from Conway and Modell's jockeyed for sidewalk space with customers walking in and out of bodegas carrying cups of coffee.

In just one day, I had gone from living in a five-bedroom house in a quiet suburb of Clarendon to a sixth-floor walkup apartment, all-day traffic jams, and a cacophony of English, Spanglish, West Indian Patois, and other languages I did not recognize. New York was a culture and lifestyle shock, and I was not ready.

As a kid, I was exposed to American culture from my siblings' stories from their visits and from watching American television shows like *The Jeffersons*, *Good Times*, and *Dynasty*. But I would soon find out that those TV shows did not come close to depicting real life in America.

I fall in the middle of six siblings, so my older brothers and sisters got to experience many things before me. My brother Garfield was allowed to visit our relatives in Florida and New York on summer holidays while we were growing up in Jamaica. He even traveled to Cincinnati to perform with our high school choir; I was never allowed on those overseas trips, except for one summer vacation trip to visit relatives in Florida. But I always fantasized about living in New York. I wanted to live in America because it seemed like a place where I could make my dreams come true.

So, there I was, finally in the USA, but my new reality was depressing. Yes, the snow was pretty and fluffy, but I sure wasn't. I hadn't ever needed a pair of gloves, a scarf, thick socks, or ugly heavy boots. I had always loved fashion and beauty, so wearing a hat over my perfectly crafted hairstyle was truly a battle between good sense and fashion sense. Same struggle over wearing a puffy jacket over my well-chosen outfits. What was even worse was having to remain cooped up in the stuffy apartment with the noisy radiator clanking away. I had to remind myself every day: I am here for a purpose.

NOT SO HUMBLE BEGINNINGS

My grandparents' home, which I'd lived in since age six, was large by Jamaican standards of the early 1970s. My grandfather owned farmland, with a decent-sized acreage in the parish of Clarendon, about a two-hour drive from Kingston in those days. My grandmother was a teacher, who, at one point, started her own school and a community and church leader. Our house was a hub for neighbors from near and far, a meeting place for the youths in the community, and a gathering spot for my father's friends, who came by to listen to music and talk politics.

Clarendon's bustling capital is called May Pen, which is anchored by the Bell Memorial Clock, a stone tower built in the early 1900s to honor a renowned doctor who died while crossing a river. Our schools were close to home, and there was a hospital and a cluster of small businesses in town. Our community of Palmer's Cross was warm and insular, green and fertile. In fact, one chore I detested most was watering the plants in the dark brown soil of my grandparents' property, where my siblings and I ran around on the cool grass after school. The river was just a short walk away, and my siblings and I swam or played community sports like soccer and netball (similar to basketball).

By the time I was in high school, our small community had grown to about sixteen homes with middle- and upper-income families of teachers, police officers, and business owners. Everybody knew everybody. We all attended the Anglican Church every Sunday, an all-day affair when you figured in Sunday School at 9:30, morning service, and then Daughters of the King in the afternoons for little girls like me. Our community youth group roped in most of the kids in the area and sponsored all sorts of civic activities. On holidays, my father and brother would set up the sound system for the entire community to listen and dance to Bob Marley, Beres Hammond, The Wailers, Gregory Isaacs, and other homegrown artists.

This was what I had known my entire life, a kind of Mayberry experience with a tropical twist. Now, here I was in big, bad New York, thinking I was going to make something of my life and not having the slightest idea how to even start.

FAMILY TREE

My big brother Garfield was always a few steps ahead of me in life. If you see me at any social event (or look at my social media pages), you will recognize him. Garfield is the dapper dude always by my side, wearing a cool hat and some fashionably expensive sneakers. He's quick with the jokes and makes everyone happy to be in the room with him. For an introvert like me, he has been an essential social lubricator. If I want to have a good time, Garfield's coming with me!

We both dreamed of being in the medical field as kids, and we achieved our goals; he is a respiratory therapist and has a doctorate in global health. In high school, Garfield was the life of the party, a star student, and popular, while I was quieter and nowhere near the top of my class. He continues to be the glue that keeps our family together. Growing up, he would spend hours talking to my grandparents about the past, our family, and Jamaica. Ask him anything about our family going back generations, and he will have the answers. (I was more concerned with my life and where it was headed.) So, I credit Garfield with a lot of the family history you will read in this book.

He is only a year and a half older than me, but he has been an inspiration, my cheerleader, and my pep-talker in chief. All his good advice, whether to finish a degree or to accept or turn down a job offer, only made my life better.

We were both very close to my father, who passed away in December of 2011. Daddy was a businessman and a politician, a deputy mayor of our town. My mother was a businesswoman as well, owning her own bar in the 1970s. My parents did not marry, although they maintained a good relationship while I was growing up. My father would go on to marry later in his life and have several other children besides my brother and me.

Living among extended family was a strong cultural tenet in my community and in Caribbean culture. Multigenerational living and caring for other people's children by taking them in as boarders were social norms. Several kids in my primary and high schools were from remote villages. Their families sent them to live nearer to the capital, Kingston, so that they could have access to better schools, and families with larger homes would take in those kids as boarders during the school week. Families like ours with working parents also would let retired or near-retired grandparents do the work of child-rearing. My grandparents had the financial means, so my mother sent us to live with them when we were quite young—Garfield as a toddler, and I went when I was about to go to basic school, or kindergarten.

WORKING MOTHER

Mommy lived about six miles away, and we saw her often. She did very well for herself and has been working ever since I have known her. Her beginnings were modest but typical for that time in the colonized Caribbean. She was one of twelve siblings from a large family in the May Pen area of Clarendon. Her house stood in a rural community: a concrete structure with just one room with a bed, table, chairs, an outdoor kitchen, and an outdoor bathroom surrounded by trees. She had another daughter, my half-sister, who was older than me and who eventually migrated to America ahead of me.

On a typical weekend, Garfield and I visited my mother, and boy, did she spoil us. Mom was one of the best cooks in our community, and she had a loyal crew who regularly came for their plates of stew peas, curry chicken, and ackee and saltfish. You name it.

I often wonder where I got my drive and ambition, and it's simple. My parents! Even though she grew up without much opportunity or access to formal education, Mommy was an industrious and savvy woman—and still is. Like me, she is relatively small, always nicely dressed, and very quiet, but she has the type of personality that draws people to her. Once she loosened up around you, she was fun to be

33

around, a great cook, and a great listener; the perfect person you want handing you a cold beer and a steaming bowl of stew peas.

Mommy's hands were always full with running her business. She was not close to my father, but she made sure that my brother and I maintained a relationship with him and his family. I think her decision showed a lot of courage, maturity, and practicality. I'm grateful that her sacrifice gave me solid emotional building blocks for a good foundation in life.

Unconsciously, I learned from my mother how to use the gifts you already have to create your own success. She used her skills as a cook and as a good listener to build a successful business where people came to her because they enjoyed her food—and her company!

Though she wasn't in our lives every day to see us off to school or ask about our homework, Mommy was and is a loving and attentive mother. As I said earlier, she was always nicely dressed and well put together, and she passed that down to me. She insisted on washing and ironing my school uniforms up until I stopped needing them in high school. The pleats in my skirt would be so neatly and crisply pressed that I would not want to sit on them.

Mommy was old-school, really old-school. When Garfield and I visited her on the weekends, she would bathe us right out in the open using what we called a bath pan, really a wide metal basin. We were between the ages of six and nine at the time. The trees kept her place private, but I was always nervous other people would see us. Mommy never cared. She bathed our little bodies and then rubbed us down with lotion. I will always remember the feel of her hands on my body; they made me feel so safe and secure.

We were a close family and continue to be. On any given Sunday, you can still find Garfield at my kitchen table on Long Island, eating my mom's rice and peas with stewed red snapper and freshly made coleslaw. We're in our fifties now, and my grandmother is long gone, but her legacy looms large over our family and our every achievement and setback. But during those first few years in the Bronx, I had to craft a life without that comforting cocoon of my community and the daily support of the extended family I had grown up with. Coming of age in the Bronx as an eighteen-year-old was challenging, like going through adolescence twice, only this time with the burden of experiencing the negative effects of race and class in America.

Life in the Boogie Down Bronx

For all the American TV I watched growing up, none of it prepared me for the pace of life in the Bronx in the 1980s. From our apartment window, I observed the pedestrians streaming every morning down the sidewalk toward the Fordham Road subway, their breath misting in the cold air. The B-Boys would drive by flexing eight-ball leather jackets, blasting KRS-One, Slick Rick, or even Shabba Ranks. Shrill sirens competed with the booming systems as Morrisania and other parts of the Bronx endured the violence and turmoil of the drug wars.

Those first few months, I spent a lot of time just looking at people, fascinated by the urgency of everything. The buses were always packed, and the drivers were always honking. From my sister and cousins, I heard the same groans: It took a lot of hard work to "make it" in New York. Most of our immigrant friends and neighbors worked at least two jobs. The rhythm of daily life was the subway to bus to work, then back again, day in and day out.

I didn't have a name for it then, but that was capitalism at the bottom: only the strong and able stood a chance of making it to the top of this impersonal system. My youth, ambition, and stamina made it easy for me to become a believer. But not everyone I knew back then became what would be described as "successful." Some of my neighbors, who worked hard and followed all the rules, remain in minimum-wage jobs and crowded, subpar apartment buildings to this day.

I knew early on that I wanted to get out of the Bronx. Even though I liked the energy of it and the familiarity of the immigrant community, the view from my window didn't square with my idea of the American dream. Where were the green grass and wide-open spaces? The spacious homes? Did these only exist on TV or in some part of the city I had yet to discover? I didn't see many people out walking or jogging for leisure or sitting at outdoor patios enjoying coffee, croissants, and a newspaper. The images I associated with having "made it" in America were not apparent to me from my corner of the Bronx.

EASY PICKINS

My older sister was a young, single mother. And she worked constantly to pay the rent and utilities and to support us. She left for America long before me, and we got along fine enough. It was her apartment, which was a real find back in those days. We had two bedrooms and enough space to spread out. I still missed the relative luxury of my grandparents' house, though. I had pictures of family, and I kept writing paper handy so I could write home—real letters on paper—to Jamaica every week or so.

But I understood that I would soon have to make my own way. I'd have to learn how to take the subway, buy clothes for each season, and learn the American currency so I wouldn't be counting change for five minutes at the store. It was overwhelming, but I was a quick learner.

Eventually, my cousin found me a minimum-wage job in Brooklyn at a store that sold candles and botanicals. The commute was long— an hour each way—for a very tiny paycheck of fifty dollars a week. I can't say I loved being in the store all day. Hardly any customers ever came in. Although I hated the smell of the candles, I was working and making money!

Keep in mind that I was barely out of my teens, so with my fifty dollars a week, I felt rich! I soon found my way to Canal Street and Delancey Road to shop for cute outfits. One of my favorite stores was Easy Pickins. The clothes were so cute, but they wouldn't survive more than one laundry cycle. And the shoes. Oh, the shoes! They would torture my poor feet. I promised myself that once I had a good job and made enough money, I would only buy clothes and shoes that were good quality.

But I was looking good and finding my way around well enough. New York was beginning to grow on me. I was falling into the rhythm of the city, rushing to the subway, unfazed by the crowds, the traffic, and the police sirens. Even the crazy scenes on the subway no longer made me stare open-mouthed.

Maybe it's because everyone moved so fast, but friends were few and far between. I mostly kept to my family, and I wrote tons of letters back home to my grandmother, my mother, and my brother Garfield, sharing with them my dreams of someday having my own apartment, becoming a nurse, and buying really nice clothes.

UNFASHIONABLY EARLY

No matter your origin country, in New York City, you're almost guaranteed to find a restaurant or a shop that has your favorite foods or music from home. On the weekends, my sister, cousins, and I would ride the bus to White Plains Road to hang out in the West Indian community. It was the closest I felt to Jamaica. The eclectic mix of storefronts, the aromas, music, and the signs along the road sparked the familiar feeling of home: patties, ackee and salt fish, and jerk everything. We could get fresh sorrel, ginger beer, black cake, rum-raisin ice cream, and reggae CDs and mixtapes from back home. And we could hear our patois being spoken in every other store we entered.

I had never been a partier; my grandmother wouldn't have stood for that. But my sister and cousins liked to get out on the weekends, so I went with them, thinking I'd finally get a chance to wear my new clothes.

The first Saturday evening they invited me out, I was dressed and sitting prim and ready to go in the living room at 7 p.m. when my cousin came out of her room wearing pajamas. "Wait! We are not going out tonight?" I asked her.

She looked me up and down, her brows creased. Slowly, my mistake dawned on her. "Girl, we don't leave here till one o'clock in the morning!"

They had a good laugh at me. One a.m.? Honestly, I didn't want to go out anymore. But I took a nap and was ready to go at 1 a.m.

Dancehall music was pounding when we entered the room, tight with bodies of girls and guys. Hands were up, and people were singing out loud as they skanked and wined to the music. It felt familiar and alien at the same time.

You would think I would just loosen up and have a good time with my people. Not so fast. I made up my mind to walk around the room and check out the vibe, so to speak. But I could almost feel my grandmother's disapproving eyes on me just for being there in the first place. I fended off guys who wanted to dance with me as kindly as I could. Why? Well, the kind of dancing at that party was not the dancing I grew up with in Palmer's Cross. People tend to think that all Jamaicans are into "wining" and grinding on the dance floor, but that is just a subculture of dancehall music. The kind of dancing I grew up with would not cause my grandmother to disown me. Needless to say, I did not enjoy clubbing that much in those days.

BUMP IN THE ROAD

Eventually, I began dating someone. He was a great guy from our circle of Jamaican friends, and we had some fun times, although I didn't think he was "the one." He surprised me in a lot of great ways then and now, including being a wonderful father to my son.

Still, life remained mainly about work and "making it." That was the constant theme of conversation in our apartment. My sister, my cousin, our friends were all working-class, striving to climb the next rung of the economic ladder. And it was a battle. At the wages we were making, buying a house was out of the question. A car was a distant possibility, maybe. But all we really wanted was a better job—to go from four dollars an hour to six dollars an hour to eight dollars an hour. That was the goal: to just be able to have something left over after paying the rent and the heat.

The American dream of the house in the suburbs, car in the garage, husband, and kids was a universe away from the reality outside our building. The Bronx in the '90s was, like many other cities at the time, in the grips of a wave of violence, with warring gangs and random shootings on a daily basis. You were happy to get inside at the end of a long workday and tune out the world outside. We kept our heads down to and from the subway and worked and worked. During that time, I don't recall any trips to the doctor for a yearly physical or even giving any thought to my health per se. I lived to work, and that was it.

I had picked up another job as a cashier at a supermarket. My commute was shorter, but, oh, how I hated that job. It wasn't the biting cold, the interminable subway rides, the panhandlers, the sirens, or the crowds that bothered me anymore. It was the slow pace of progress. I had been in America for nearly three years, and I was earning four dollars an hour, standing on my feet all day, and being subject to insults and abuse from some of the rudest customers. One day, a man came up to my aisle and threw his basket of groceries onto the belt.

"Sir," I asked him. "Could you please remove the groceries first?"

He glared at me. "What's wrong with your hands?" he growled.

At that point, I could have cried; I felt my life was going nowhere. My mom had just moved to New York, and together, we were renting a two-bedroom apartment. My brother Garfield was going to be joining us soon from Jamaica, and I would soon find out that I was pregnant.

Looking back now as a health-care executive, I can see my young self as a case study. Oh, the encouragement I would give that young girl if I could just go back! But I was just a kid then, trying my very best to survive and overcome my circumstances.

Most nights, I would stumble into bed in tears. I was so ashamed of what my grandmother would think if she saw me pregnant, unmarried, and working as a cashier in a grocery store. I wanted to quit that job so badly, but I didn't. I couldn't. I had bills to pay and a baby on the way.

CHAPTER 6

Privilege to Pauper: My Father

R ecently, I was at work in a patient's room and my picture popped up on the TV. He gave me a second glance, looking at my nametag, and recognition dawned on his face. No, it wasn't from my vaccine advocacy work. He actually knew me.

"I know her father from back in Jamaica!" the patient exclaimed. "They're big time where they come from. Everybody knows the Lindsay family." As I joked with the man about life in Jamaica, I could see that other people in the room were looking at me with a question in their eyes. To them, I was just Sandra the nurse, the director of the ICU, not someone linked by blood to a well-known Jamaican politician.

MY FATHER, THE HERO

Around Father's Day in 2023, I began to think about my father, missing him in a way I hadn't in a long time. In the days leading up to that

Sunday, I'd been teary-eyed and feeling down, not my normal self at all. My life was busy with events, speaking at graduations, appearing on health-related podcasts, plus maintaining my full-time job. Maybe it was exhaustion, or maybe COVID-19 grief was finally catching up to me. I wracked my brain for the reason, but couldn't figure out why I was so despondent. On that Sunday while in the shower, long suppressed memories began to flood my mind.

My father was a charismatic man who loved Jamaica. He was short, had a dark complexion, and had a beer belly. But he was very popular among the ladies. He moved to the US in the 1990s but only lived here for a few years before returning home. My father wasn't the sort to just talk about changing things in our community; he believed in acting on his convictions. He was a serious man, and because of that, my siblings were a little afraid of him. Not me, though. My siblings will tell you that I was my father's favorite. They would probably exaggerate: I could get anything I wanted. I was spoiled. I will admit that my father and I were especially close. He loved music, and I will always remember the absolute joy playing music brought him. We had a music sound system called Global Hi-Fi, which my oldest brother, Dave, managed until he died of cancer at the young age of thirty. But this was one of my father's favorite things to do—set up the Global HiFi with his son Dave and play music for our entire community to gather around and enjoy.

Growing up, I always felt safe in my grandparents' home. There was a time when the wall around the house was barely three feet high. You could just walk over it. The fence was more decorative than anything. Now, however, the wall is ten feet high and completely surrounds the house with locked gates. There is also a sophisticated security system. These security measures are quite a contrast from my days as a kid and a young teen when we never even had bars on the windows.

The security was well justified. As I described earlier, my father had been a political target, plus the crime rate in Jamaica had been steadily rising each year. We were not immune.

INTRUDER

One night, I was sleeping with my grandmother in her room because my grandfather was away at his farm in the country. I must have been an adolescent then.

I was sleeping soundly when I suddenly sensed a shadow was over me. I opened my eyes and saw a person with a towel over their head and holding out a knife at my neck. I screamed as loud as I could. The person ran away, jumping back out of the bathroom window they had broken in through. My poor grandmother and I were terrified. I was frozen in fear, and she was in no condition to run after the intruder.

I could hardly speak. Was this person coming to really kill me? I panicked. Why and who would do something like that? We never did find out who the intruder was that night.

But soon, my father and his friends were at the house, and I felt so much safer and comforted by his presence. By the next day, my father had welders making grills to cover every window and had reinforced every type of security measure he could around the house. My father went to work immediately to make sure his family was safe. I imagine he did a lot more that I didn't know about or could have understood at that age. But what I do remember is the sense of security of seeing him there, working with his hands to make sure I was safe.

DANGEROUS POLITICS

When I was about eleven or twelve, my father was shot, and it wouldn't be the only time. I had just started high school at the time, and it was a terrible two-year period in my life. Just a year later, I was infected with Dengue fever and was very sick for several months. The political trouble with my father had long been brewing, and his life had been threatened quite a few times.

During Jamaica's political turmoil of the 1980s, my father was a leader in our parish, Clarendon, as a counselor and a deputy mayor. My father was well-respected and loved by the several constituencies under his leadership. But there were opponents, and they were loud and violent. Many lived nearby and had names and faces we could easily identify. As the threats increased, he never once considered stepping down from his position. During the elections in 1980, the tension had grown so bad that my father was shot several times on several occasions. They were non-life-threatening injuries, but it was terrifying, probably the biggest event in my relatively normal and sheltered childhood.

What my father's courage meant for me as a kid was fear. At first, my siblings and I were not too sure why there were men guarding our house at times. We were used to having Daddy's friends around, so we chalked it up to that. But one year during election season, I learned the truth in a way that would turn me off politics for the rest of my life.

Garfield and I walked to the neighborhood store to collect our weekly groceries every Saturday. It was part of our weekly routine. One day, we walked our same route to the store, playing and joking the entire way. We were eleven and twelve at the time. This was a small shop that sold candy and grocery items, a place where the community shopped and socialized. We didn't pay too much attention to the group of young guys hanging outside the store; we continued to approach the store, oblivious to the looks that were coming our way.

We didn't slow down until we heard one of them shout out something to the effect of:

"Those are his children!"

The guys began to come toward us quickly, with menacing looks on their faces.

"Run!" I heard either from me or from Garfield, and run is what we did as quickly as our legs would go. We sprinted from the store and across long-abandoned train tracks, running through our town until we burst into my grandparents' house, scared out of our minds and panting for breath.

That incident made clear to me what my father was involved in as a community leader. This was serious business. We found out that my father sent a message to the gang leading the charge to hurt us that if they ever laid hands on us, they would suffer the consequences of their actions. Needless to say, that was the end of supporting the local grocery store in that area, which we preferred going to over the big-box supermarkets.

Despite my father's anger over this incident, he continued to serve his constituents and took more safety measures. We now had twenty-four-hour guards at the house. We were not allowed to go to school during that or other election seasons.

There were hushed conversations about new threats to my father, and those conversations would abruptly stop when we kids entered the room. If we were caught in certain areas, we would be killed, was the message from my father's enemies. It was a hostile, volatile time.

One night, I woke up to more commotion in our house. Some of the young guys from the other party had poured gasoline around the house to set it ablaze. Luckily, the perpetrators were stopped before they could do any real harm, but there was no sleeping the rest of that night and for many afterward.

You might be asking why these things were happening. In my opinion, these political fights were simply about obtaining power, and there was no noble objective other than who would get access and power. The people who targeted our family were young guys, people we knew as neighbors in the grocery store and from school, but that's what politics did to communities in those days. My grandmother, who had taught some of these young boys in school, pleaded with them to stop the threats and the intimidation, but they only shrugged.

"Sorry. It's politics, and we do what we have to do for our party."

Through it all, my father continued to serve, even though serving his community put him in mortal danger.

I can't say that I inherited my father's courage. I have been fortunate that, with all the public outrage around the vaccine debate, I have never received a single threat. And besides the terrible events of January 6, 2021, I have never experienced in America the horrible violence that I witnessed as a child growing up in Jamaica. And I am so grateful for that.

If I had just a fraction of my father's courage, I'd count myself lucky. When I think of what he went through, it inspires me to serve selflessly

46

and without fear! My father was a brave man who must have learned from his courageous and selfless mother, my grandmother, that it is worth it to take a risk to make a difference in people's lives.

MY FATHER'S HUMILITY

In addition to being a politician, my father was a successful businessman who owned a shopping plaza for a time. But eventually, his businesses failed. That happened a few years after I had left for America, and I did not have a first-hand look at how my father experienced losing his businesses and eventually quitting politics. I imagine it had to have been difficult for him emotionally.

In the 1990s, my father emigrated to America. He was in his late fifties but was still up for another challenge: to take advantage of the economic opportunities the US offered. By that time, he had married and had three more children.

While my father was well-known and respected in Jamaica, when he came to America, he was an unknown, just another immigrant working low-wage jobs. He humbled himself to take these jobs in America, adapting to the social and economic hierarchy despite all he had accomplished in his own country. America was a culture shock for my father. He would say: Oh, my God! This is what America is like? But he stuck it out because my younger siblings needed him to provide for them.

I thought of my father not only as a leader and a provider but as a protector. One childhood incident sticks out in my memory.

If my father was suffering from losing his status in America, one would never know. He always kept his dignity about him because he was providing for his family every step of the way. He left his privilege behind and became a pauper as a Black immigrant in America. His humility and persistence taught me resilience and imbued me with the courage to fight for what I believe in.

Eventually, he returned to Jamaica. I am so glad he was able to go back to Jamaica and live the life of dignity and respect that he had worked so hard for his entire life. Thankfully, he did not die a pauper in America, but as the proud Jamaican statesman he had been his entire life.

CHAPTER 7

Privilege to Pauper: My Weekend in the Hamptons

S ometimes we bury painful incidents in our lives just so we can move forward, but then an unearthing occurs, making the ground underneath you a little shaky. It could be a movie, a book, or just a person on the street that triggers a memory, and those feelings come rushing back. That happened to me around Father's Day recently when I could not get my father out of my mind, and childhood memories flooded my mind for several days. Reliving past experiences, especially the sad ones, can be complicated, even detrimental. Later in the book, I will talk more about the "weathering" health effects of living in an unjust society and how that can affect marginalized people.

I had one of those triggering moments recently as I read Linda Villarosa's *Under the Skin*. Villarosa, a health-care journalist, has done some valuable work on the discrimination and inequity prevalent in health-care setting, particularly relating to maternal and black women's health care. Her book stirred up the most painful memories of my own pregnancy and birthing experience, which I describe in a later chapter.

I have not lived my entire life in America. But I can only imagine the painful stories told in the households of African Americans who have had many more years to accumulate incidents of bias, hostility, and even outright violence. These incidents can be destructive in the moment and later on when the cumulative effects over the years cause harm to our mind, body, and soul.

Racial mistreatment was not something I planned for or even considered when I arrived in America. I came to America to pursue my dream of becoming a nurse and making my family proud. I honestly did not think that my status as an immigrant and a young Black woman could, in isolation, seriously impact my life, but it did.

LUCKY ME

When I was finally ready for my big move from Jamaica, my father gave me fifty dollars for the trip to America for spending money. In those days, you had to go to the bank to buy American dollars, and so that's what I did. What a day that was! I felt so important as I entered the air-conditioned bank with my passport and ticket in hand. There, I showed them, I was indeed going to live in America! My hopes were soaring when I walked out of that bank with fifty US dollars in my purse. I was so lucky to have family sponsorship for my visa and a place to live in New York. During that time of political and economic turmoil in Jamaica, every other person wanted to leave for the US or the United Kingdom.

Besides that first job in the botanicals shop in Brooklyn, I took on other odd jobs those first few years in the Bronx. I would scour the classified ads in the *New York Post* on Sundays, searching for babysitting and other jobs that didn't require a degree: cashier, babysitter, and then some.

One Sunday, I saw this job advertised: a weekend to go to the Hamptons and prepare a home for the summer. "Wow," I thought. "Just a weekend? I can do that and keep my weekday job!" From the babysitting circuit, I knew that if a person had a house in the Hamptons, they had to be a multimillionaire. And if they could afford to pay for help, well, it had to be a nice house. Sounded like a nothing-to-lose deal to me!

I called the number and scheduled the interview. It was with a well-known physician at a major hospital in the city. She and her family needed some extra help to get their summer house ready, she said, nothing too heavy. The conversation went great, although a bit impersonal. But it would be seventy-five dollars a day, she promised, for some cleaning up and organizing. Of course, I gladly accepted the job.

My weekend in the Hamptons with this family started out well enough. We all packed up in a station wagon, with the husband and wife in the front and their huge fluffy dog, their luggage, and me in the backseat. When the fluffy dog began to lean on me, I began to question my decision, but the thought of seventy-five dollars a day kept me on board. We finally pulled up to this lavish house in the Hamptons. Yes, it was a gorgeous neighborhood with massive homes spaced far apart. At that point in my life, I wasn't too impressed by the beauty of the Hamptons, however. Nothing could compare with my beloved Jamaica when it came to natural beauty. But, yes, it was a beautiful (although a little too manicured) beach town.

SOME LIGHT WORK

So, there I was in the Hamptons, ready to work. I should mention that, in those days, I weighed barely a hundred pounds at five foot four. The couple put me to work immediately and disappeared.

From early morning till late into the night on Friday, I worked, cleaning and dusting, washing clothes, and basically housekeeping in this dusty mansion that had been locked up for months. My living and sleeping quarters were this tiny attic room with a slanted roof that I could barely stand in.

The couple then announced there was a dinner on Saturday night that I wasn't invited to. Surprise! I began early that Saturday at the main house, cleaning, preparing for the party, and chopping what seemed like thousands of peppers for this fancy dinner. On Saturday afternoon, I found myself pushing a wheelbarrow, moving lawn clippings, and moving dirt. Definitely not the light work—vacuuming, dusting—I expected.

I stopped at one point to consider what I was doing: If my grandmother saw me pushing this wheelbarrow, she would kill me! Here I was, this girl who grew up in relative privilege in Jamaica, being treated like an invisible person by this wealthy family. I say invisible person because that's what they seemed to want from me: to work and to disappear. I would eat in my attic room and then come out to work. It was a strange feeling for me—to be completely disregarded as a person and treated as a unit of production.

While working in their yard, I remembered the people my grandmother hired to help her around the house. We knew each of these men and women by name. While they worked in our home, we talked with them, and they ate with us at mealtime, and there was mutual respect.

Boy, was I naive! There was so much I didn't know about life in America. But that weekend, I began to learn, for example, how wealth, ethnicity, education, or the lack thereof, created distance between people and were used as tools to elevate and diminish folks.

My employers that weekend, despite our chatty, friendly drive from New York City to East Hampton in their car with their fluffy dog, could decide to just stop *seeing* me once we arrived at their summer house and their Hamptons persona took over. I just no longer existed for them, it seemed. The mental shift is mind-boggling to me even now when I recall how naturally and quickly this shift happened for them.

Back in Jamaica, I had never pushed a wheelbarrow in my life because, in my family, that type of work was reserved for men. But what could I do? I willingly signed up for this job that would pay me seventy-five dollars a day, which I desperately needed.

The weekend ended, finally. Exhausted and relieved to be going home, I was excited for the $225 coming to me. I had already planned what I would do with it—pay my bills. Plus, I really needed to get those Jheri curls done.

On Sunday evening, when I was ready to leave, the wife handed me a check for seventy-five dollars. I looked up at her in confusion. "This is a mistake," I said. "I thought it was seventy-five dollars a day." She shook her head no. "It's seventy-five dollars for the weekend. I could have gotten it done for fifty dollars!" She was already angry, and I hadn't even raised my voice.

I was so shocked and disappointed that I could only look away from this woman who had suddenly become so intimidating and scary. She went back into the house after letting me know that her husband would drive me back to the city while the rest of them remained in the Hamptons. I had no words, no protest, no ground to stand on. It was my mistake, according to her, and I had to live with it.

What made everything worse was the long, silent ride back to New York City. I cried the entire way, hoping the husband didn't see my tears. I was dropped off at the subway station, where I would travel back to the Bronx.

SPEAKING ON IT

For years, I had stuffed this incident deep down in a closet of shame. Just the memory of it triggers so much anger. I did not want to include it in this book. I thought if anyone ever knew that I went through this... But wait, I stopped myself. What had I done wrong? Why should I feel shame for the despicable behavior of these people? It was they who should feel shame at taking advantage of my naivete and powerlessness. And if they don't, then that says a lot about their lack of humanity. And just like that, I began to feel empowered. What had I done wrong except go out and work very hard and expect to be paid fairly for my labor?

Many people—immigrants, the poor, minorities—likely can recall similar incidents in their lives. Many of us were taken advantage of economically or in other ways and then made to feel shame if we dared to stand up for ourselves. We might have even been threatened to keep silent in the face of mistreatment. As a young immigrant just one year in America, I believed I could do nothing but cower in shame and hope the rich husband didn't see my tears. Today, I am telling this family and anyone who treats other people this way that they should feel shame for mistreating the poor and powerless. Such attitudes are so cancerous to our society.

I was in church recently, and the preacher was talking about his experience growing up poor but pulling himself up with hard work to live a comfortable life in Jamaica. Then, he emigrated to America only to be treated like a pauper again. He recounted living paycheck to paycheck, not being able to afford rent, and moving multiple times. It was a familiar story: the disorienting sense of loss of the comfortable and familiar, of having to rebuild yourself from scratch in a country where nobody knows your name and they're not always glad you came.

My pastor called it the "privilege to pauper" experience. My experience in the Hamptons that weekend in 1987 was one of the many pauper moments I would have in America.

CHAPTER 8

My First Virus

T he Jamaica of my childhood was tranquil, green, and orderly. My grandparents tried to protect my siblings and me from the outside world, and they did a really good job. As a small child, I was mostly unaware of the political upheaval plaguing our capital, Kingston, in the 1970s. Three headlines from the *New York Times* in 1976 illustrate the turmoil that had gained international attention: "Jamaica Worried by Slum Fighting" from January 8, 1976; "Fear in Paradise" from July 25, 1976—an opinion piece that described Jamaica as "an angry, insecure third-world state with an almost bankrupt economy that barely supports its two million citizens"—and "Choice for Jamaicans: Ties With Third or Whole World" from November 29, 1976.[15]

---

[15] Edward Cowan, "Choice for Jamaicans: Ties with Third or Whole World," *New York Times*, November 29, 1976, https://www.nytimes.com/1976/11/29/archives/choice-for-jamaicans-ties-with-third-or-whole-world.html.

Stephen Davis, "Fear in Paradise," *New York Times*, July 25, 1976, https://www.nytimes.com/1976/07/25/archives/fear-in-paradise-the-real-jamaica-is-an-angry-state-locked-in-a.html.

On December 15, 1976, Jamaicans reelected the socialist People's Nationalist Party back to power. The US was interested (probably an understatement) as the PNP's leader, Michael Manley, had been steadily strengthening his ties with Cuba and extolling the value of socialism. In Jamaica, most of the wealth was owned and controlled by White, Chinese, Lebanese, and Syrian Jamaicans, and the bauxite industry was controlled by US and British companies. The more conservative Jamaica Labor Party had been the first to lead Jamaica after it claimed independence from Great Britain in 1962. The Labor Party accused the PNP of stoking anti-White and pro-Communist sentiment. Leading up to that 1976 election, political violence claimed hundreds of lives, left entire communities torched, and caused many native-born and expatriate Whites and Asians to flee the country, fearing that their property would be seized or that they would face violence from the poor people living in the slums of Kingston. It was also during that time that attempts were made on Bob Marley's life. We lived far enough away from the capital and the terror that gripped West Kingston and the poorer areas of the capital. But eventually, the political mood in the country did touch my family years later as I described in the previous chapter.

ELECTION SEASON MEANT STAYING IN

The shooting attack on my father was a non-life-threatening injury, but it was terrifying, probably the biggest event in my relatively normal and sheltered childhood. The fear and anxiety in our household and community around elections remain with me to this day. What that meant for my life was staying home from school, lessons from my grandmother, and playing endless board games with my siblings. Those were the times when I would observe Garfield sidling up to my grandparents and asking

---

Leonard Silk, "Jamaica Worried by Slum Fighting," *New York Times*, January 8, 1976, https://www.nytimes.com/1976/01/08/archives/jamaica-worried-by-slum-fighting-outburst-in-kingston-while-imf.html.

For a wonderfully written fictionalized account of this time in Jamaica, read Marlon James's *A Brief History of Seven Killings*, published in 2014 by Riverhead Books.

them all kinds of questions about our family history. I didn't care enough to eavesdrop for long; I just hated being inside. My grandmother did her best to keep us distracted. She tried to teach us how to play the organ, and I did my best not to learn it! Oh, how I envied the neighborhood kids I could see from my window, playing outside, going to school, to the river, and living their carefree lives.

To this day, I am traumatized and not a big fan of politics. I do care deeply about global current events but mostly about how the less powerful and less fortunate are mistreated by some power-hungry, corrupt politicians. The political and economic conditions of Jamaica were precarious, and tens of thousands of people were leaving for the UK and the United States as soon as they could get their hands on a visa. Our family members soon began to think about emigration.

INSECURE TEENAGE YEARS

I graduated from Jamaica's elite Glenmuir High School. Glenmuir is built on a leafy, beautiful campus and patterned on the British educational system. We had the regular high school rivalries over sports, academics, school clubs (we called them houses), and girlfriends and boyfriends. There was every activity you could think of: choir, sports, national quiz competition. Like the community I grew up in, it was safe and comfortable. Our teachers were well-educated, and they took their jobs seriously. There was an air of dignity about everything at Glenmuir.

My brother Garfield was popular on campus, sang in the school choir, and was loved by everyone. It didn't help that I was a transfer student, and by the time I came, a lot of the cliques were formed, and it was hard to find my place. I was so quiet, and hardly anyone knew I was Garfield's sister. I tended to stay closer to home and hung out with the same two to three girls for most of high school. Garfield, on the other hand, will admit that he had a different experience as a boy growing up in Jamaica. He was allowed to travel across the country and overseas with his friends, camping, hanging out, or performing in the choir. I was always close to home. I won't attribute Garfield's relative freedom to sexism or anything like that, although there was an element of tradition in the way boys and girls were raised in Jamaica in those days.

I wasn't among what you would call the popular girls. My high school reflected the wider Jamaican society at the time and was sharply stratified by color, an embarrassing and shameful remnant of colonialism.[16] I was a dark-skinned girl with hair and features that were far from European, and unfortunately, I did not always see myself as beautiful. I always felt insecure with my looks as a teenager, and I experimented a lot with different hairstyles and makeup, trying to find the perfect look, a practice that actually taught me a lot about makeup and hair. To this day, I enjoy shopping and getting my makeup and hair done professionally, although I can admit that I do a pretty bang-up job on myself. And thankfully, today, when I look in the mirror, I love the gorgeous woman looking back at me!

UNWELCOME GUEST

In my second year of high school, I mysteriously began to lose weight. I would wake up in sweats, spiking a fever, and feeling very weak. I didn't know what was wrong with me, but each time I looked in the mirror, my body seemed to be disappearing. At five foot four, I was often called skinny, and I absolutely hated it. As you can imagine, the sudden additional weight loss was frightening and distressing.

Sickness was always hovering over my life, it seemed. My grandmother suffered from diabetes and hypertension, and taking care of her was always part of my life. My siblings and I took turns going to doctor's appointments with her and helping her with her medications. One of my mother's sisters died from ovarian cancer when she was quite young. I may have been around nine at the time, and I saw her fight the illness

---

16   Some Americans are shocked when they hear Jamaican Patois spoken by blond-haired, blue-eyed whites and Asians. But Jamaica has always had a diverse population made up of descendants of African slaves, indentured workers, and Lebanese and Syrians who immigrated to the islands in the nineteenth century. Even with all this diversity, dark-skinned people remained at the bottom of the social, economic, and political hierarchy.

and grow weaker, shrinking every time we went to visit. Several years later, my oldest brother David would die of stomach cancer while he was only in his thirties.

For months, I was in bed, out of school, away from my regular life and the few friends that I had, with fevers that wouldn't break and debilitating weakness. Still, I thought sickness was for older people. I was just a kid, and it would pass. The weakness in my body left me unable to play, unable to go outside and run around in the garden, and unable to concentrate on schoolwork. Back and forth to the doctor we went for months. My poor grandmother! My mother was worried, of course. She was hands-on, treating me like a baby again, bathing me, and attending to my every need. My siblings tried to make life as normal for me as possible by keeping me up to date on the school gossip, and my grandmother made sure I never missed a lesson by teaching me at home. I was stuck inside and was too weak to go even a short distance.

There was a huge mango tree in our backyard, and I could go out there some days. This was where Garfield and I would sit and talk, dreaming out loud. My father would joke that we were plotting against the other siblings. But we were only talking about the futures we wanted. I wanted to be a nurse, and Garfield wanted to be a doctor. As our older siblings began to emigrate abroad, we continued to dream of a better life for ourselves overseas as well.

We talked about traveling to faraway countries, even down to what we would wear on the plane. My grandmother bought us several books that exposed us to cultures all over the world, like India, the Philippines, and countries in Africa. The nuggets of information we gathered about those countries would spark a curiosity in us. We would say: "Oh, this place looks so interesting. I want to go there when I grow up." And, sure enough, Garfield and I did grow up to visit many of those countries.

But dreaming under the mango tree did not shorten my bout with sickness. Visits to the doctor's office in May Pen were tedious; it wasn't the place any kid wanted to go. We had very few doctors for the population size, and this one doctor that my family trusted with my health was everybody's doctor. His office was very busy. It took several visits before I was finally diagnosed with Dengue fever.

NATIONAL OUTBREAK

Dengue fever is spread by mosquitoes and causes fevers, rashes, and aches and pains. More serious strains can include hemorrhagic fever and even death. In 1977, a Dengue outbreak was sweeping across the Caribbean and even to some states in the US, infecting tens of thousands of people in several countries and sixty thousand in Jamaica alone.[17]

The 1977 dengue outbreak is just one vivid illustration of the impact of health-care disparities on a global scale. The Jamaican primary health system made successful efforts to educate the population about dengue and preventive measures. Research[18] showed that information about the virus was broadcast on radio and television to towns and villages.

Yet, a majority of respondents to a survey of rural Westmoreland Parish acknowledged that while they had been educated about dengue transmission, they did not use effective dengue preventive methods, such as screening of homes or using bed nets. In that same research report, the authors noted that Jamaica's response to dengue outbreaks had been largely reactionary, meaning that officials took action after dengue had already established itself in the population. The report attributed Jamaica's limited response to budgetary cutbacks and resource constraints. For example, there was only one "poorly equipped" lab that could test for dengue on the island, and there were insufficient funds to undertake an adequate vector control program—such as spraying insecticides in affected areas.

I know of many Jamaicans who did not have the money for medicines or doctor visits. For people who lived far away from Montego Bay

---

[17] "Dengue Fever Outbreak Reported in Jamaica; 2 U.S. Cases Suspect," *New York Times*, July 17, 1977, https://www.nytimes.com/1977/07/17/archives/dengue-fever-outbreak-reported-in-jamaica-2-us-cases-suspect.html.

[18] Faisal Shuaib et al., "Knowledge, Attitudes and Practices Regarding Dengue Infection in Westmoreland, Jamaica," *West Indian Medical Journal*, 59, 2 (2010): 139–46, https://www.ncbi.nlm.nih.gov/pmc/articles/PMC2996104/.

and Kingston, where one went for care when village or local doctors couldn't provide the care needed, serious illness meant long journeys on poor roads. Similarly, on the smaller islands in the Eastern Caribbean, it was common for very sick people (who had the means) to travel to Jamaica, Barbados, or Trinidad and Tobago to get treatment for major diseases or to have complicated surgeries. That need for "health-care tourism" continues to this day in the Caribbean. But back then, even the best hospitals in Kingston and Montego Bay lacked many of the services and resources that were common in hospitals in the UK and the US.

For poor children in a developing country, dengue fever can mean unnecessary suffering and long-term ill health, even death. If parents are not able to afford a doctor who can advise them how to properly manage the illness, the results can be dire. For some kids, it could mean the end of their education. They might miss a few weeks, months, or a year of school or just never return.

I was fortunate to have been in a supportive, economically stable environment. My grandmother gave me school lessons at home during those months when I couldn't attend school. My mother was there every day to bathe me, feed me, and take me to doctors' appointments. The constant trips to the doctor and the medicines cost money, all paid for by my grandparents. The doctor I saw during my illness was a familiar figure in our community. He was kind to me and my grandmother, and we felt comfortable with him and the other caregivers. Even in a country where access to adequate health-care services was in short supply, having caring doctors and a supportive, stable family made up for a lot of what was lacking.

In later chapters, we will see that in America, inequities in health care can have the same outcomes for the poor and marginalized here as those in developing countries despite America's vast wealth and advanced health-care system.

CHAPTER 9

Teenage Angst

High school was thirty-eight years ago! That fact really hit home when I delivered the commencement address virtually to Glenmuir's graduating class of 2021. It's been nearly forty years since I was a student, not knowing how my life would turn out. Over the years, I've attended reunions at Glenmuir on a couple of occasions, and each time, it has been a joy to walk through those classrooms and see my teachers and former classmates. While attending Glenmuir, I didn't think anyone even knew my name, but that was not true then, and it certainly isn't true now. All those childish feelings of insecurity are where they belong—in the past. I am enjoying getting to see my classmates in this phase of life, as parents and grandparents, movers and shakers, people who effect change on our island, in the world, and in their families. I will go back as often as I can, and I will always be proud to have been part of the class of 1985.

Like most high schools in the caribbean at that time, you had to successfully complete an admission exam to get into high school. There were brilliant kids from poor backgrounds who had passed their subjects and were doing very well in school. Some boarded at my grandparents' house. That stood in contrast to the rich kids who were born into the pipeline of the best elementary and primary schools that led them to Glenmuir. Their drivers dropped them off and picked them up from school every day. Some even had their own cars. Their parents—politicians, industry executives, landowners, expatriates—had national influence, so everyone knew their names. Those kids were more extroverted and confident and had hundreds of friends.

You might be familiar with the colorism conversation. Growing up in Jamaica, it was not talked about, but colorism was entrenched and, dare I say, accepted in the Jamaica I grew up in. Jamaica has a diverse population in terms of phenotypes and ethnic background: we have Jamaicans of European descent, blond-haired and blue-eyed, whose family lines go back hundreds of years on the island and whose Jamaican accent is thicker than mine. We have Chinese, Indian, and Middle Eastern Jamaicans who also have been on the island for generations. From the 1930s, a number of Syrians and Lebanese began to move to the Caribbean islands and settled there, opening businesses and forming a strong middle and upper class. In addition, some Asians were brought as indentured workers and remained as citizens at all levels of Jamaican society. Some descendants of British slaveowners and other European members of the plantation economy never left the island. There has always been a range of skin colors, hair types, and so forth on the island. And this doesn't even include the native population, which includes Taino and Arawak peoples who originated in South America before Columbus arrived.

I can only talk about my experience. But take my word for it that as a dark-skinned black girl, I felt devalued in school, particularly in my high school, which was largely populated by middle- and upper-class kids who tended to have lighter skin. It didn't help that I lacked confidence to begin with and always tried to hide myself, especially when dating and relationships became more important in school life.

SCHOOL DAZE

In primary school, I mostly kept to myself. I was concerned with follow-ing my grandmother's rules, and she did not encourage playing around with boys. In high school, that began to change as I began to see cute boys I liked. However, I never felt that any boy could like me. The girls who were getting the most attention had lighter skin and smoother hair than me. I felt ashamed that I wasn't as pretty and as wanted as those girls. I had two close friends in high school, and to this day, I value the friendship we had; we stuck close together, and that helped me survive some of the teenage angst years. One passed away a few years ago, and I want to honor her memory here by just being grateful for her friendship throughout my life.

My brother, who is also dark-skinned, didn't have this problem. As an active member of the school choir, he was always very popular and socially active, while I sort of stood back in the shadows. Looking back now, I see that I could have been a bit more outgoing. I could have shared my sparkling personality, sense of humor, and authentic self with my friends. My lack of confidence came largely from the stories I was telling myself, and those stories were not based on truth at all! I would learn later on in life that many of us in high school were struggling in our own ways, and I was far from alone.

To make it worse, I wasn't doing that great academically. As I dis-cussed earlier, I had a serious bout of dengue fever, which took me out of school for months, leaving me behind in some classes. Insecurity was just firing at me from every angle. I knew even then that I wanted to be a nurse, but I was so discouraged about underperforming in my subjects! It seemed that everyone around me was beautiful, athletic, and a genius.

These are difficult things—colorism, shame, insecurity—for a teen-ager to deal with, even for adults to talk about. Reflecting on my strug-gles helps me to empathize with our younger generation, who, in some ways, are worse off because of the constant pressure from social media.

Thankfully, I'm no longer that scared, insecure teen. But I also know that my experience is not unique and that even the girls who I thought were so beautiful and had it all also experienced insecurities about their looks and felt unsure of themselves in some way.

All of us, especially women, must face those uncomfortable feelings about ourselves, even though they might unearth shame and anger. The earlier we deal with those feelings and emotions, the better, because the longer we let them fester, the more they take root and sprout into negative thought patterns and behavior, preventing us from enjoying and experiencing the fullness that life has to offer. Whether it is through therapy, faith practice, or whatever other healthy methods, please do not let negative and shameful wrong thinking dominate your life. Make it a priority to silence and kill those lying voices for good!

YOU ARE BEAUTIFUL

I wish I could speak to my younger self now and tell her how beautiful she was and how she should not have hidden herself or felt any shame about her looks. Clearly, I was wrong because other people saw my beauty.

I was sixteen when he first approached me; we knew each other from our community, but he had graduated years before me. He was a dream to look at, tall and handsome. But he was half-Syrian and had a lighter complexion and smooth textured hair. I was intimidated and smitten the first time he even said hello to me. My shyness did not deter him.

Why would he like me so much that he would drive by the school every day at closing to offer me a ride home? His attention always confused me. Everyone knew him and his family, and he could have probably any girl he wanted. Again, with my insecurities leading the way like the band in a parade, I laid my self-doubts bare to this poor guy. I asked him straight out one day, "Why do you like me?" His answer was simple. He thought I was beautiful, he said. He liked my dark skin.

But did I believe him? Come on!

He did his best to reassure me, and I give him kudos—how many older guys would do this today? He wrote me long letters in cursive, telling me how much he cared about me, calling me his "African Princess."

64

Around him, I was always "beautiful this" or "beautiful that." And, no, it wasn't a scheme to get fresh with me. This young man drove to our property in Palmer's Cross to ask my father whether he could date me. I stood in the living room, embarrassed and a little afraid my father would embarrass him. He spoke like someone definitely older than his years and probably a bit too ambitious for where we were in life as teenagers. He wanted to take care of me, he told my father.

My father shrugged it off. But this young man followed the rules to a T. When he visited our house, we would sit on the veranda in sight of everyone. The rule was we could date as long as we stayed out in the open, and so we did.

I should have felt special, loved, beautiful. This could have been the great love of my life. I wasn't one for romance novels or movies, but I wanted to feel loved and adored by a handsome man, as many girls my age did. But did I just sit back and bask in the attention? Nope. I doubted him and myself constantly. I wondered out loud what he possibly could see in me. It didn't help that his family was cold toward me when he proudly brought me to his family events. Certain members of his family would not even look at me. Their coldness only added another layer to my insecurities.

But this was such a good guy. He never gave up. He would pick me up from school and drive me around our town proudly. I was more afraid to be seen with him than anything; I thought people would laugh at me for thinking that such a good-looking guy would want to be with me. Eventually, we grew apart, and I moved away, but I still think of him.

What a missed opportunity! What unnecessary pain I inflicted on myself!

SPEAKING OF UNNECESSARY PAIN

As much as we can long for the music of the '90s or the simplicity and freedom of the '80s, there are some things we want to remain at the bottom of the dustbin of history. I'm talking about entire Saturdays spent at the hairdressers getting Vaselined and then permed and burned, only to do it all again six weeks later.

I begged my mother and grandmother to please let me have a perm when I was eleven or twelve. Begged. My hair was too thick. I couldn't handle it. Blah Blah. I broke them down, and they eventually gave in to my whining. I then began my self-imposed life sentence of permed and processed hair. I only granted myself parole when I realized a few years ago that it had been decades since I had seen or touched my natural hair! Decades.

The truth was, in my high school, my tight curls were not considered beautiful or attractive. Before hitting my teens, I had the idea ingrained in my head that my natural, God-given hair was not acceptable or beautiful. What a way to begin life as an adolescent! Over the years, I have had my hair adventures, journeys, struggles, and epiphanies. I've had my hair fall out during an illness. I've had to fire or break up with bad hairdressers. I've had good ones who really, really hooked me up. Some mornings, I look in the mirror and decide it's just going to have to be a scarf day.

I'm coming to the realization that what I really want out of my hair is to be able to love it, to touch it, and to revel in its natural beauty. That's what I want—I'm not fully there yet. My "hair journey" will probably continue as long as I live, but I'm glad to at least be moving in the right direction. Legislation like the Crown Act, which protects against discrimination against natural hair in the workplace and other settings, is a milestone our youth initiated and should be praised for pursuing. I'm ecstatic when I see Gen Zers and Millennials walking about so freely with their natural hair out in locs, braids, cornrows, fros, and everything in between. Seeing news anchors, corporate executives, and doctors embracing their natural hair is one of the blessings of living in this particular time in our society. It's wonderful for me to meet a young lady who has never had the misfortune of encountering a relaxer, who has never had a scalp burn from lye. It is amazing to walk through a CVS in Manhattan or Long Island and see products on the shelves for Black natural hair. This is not the 1980s, and I am here for it!

LOVING OUR ENTIRE SELVES

Whether because of our skin color, our weight, our hair, or whatever ridiculous arbitrary standard society has set, many of us are blind to our beauty, and this blindness dulls our other senses. We miss out on opportunities to love ourselves and to experience the love of others.

My teenage relationship was very precious to me, even though I may have screwed it up with my self-doubt and insecurities. But I learned so much from it once I had the maturity to reflect on my role and my missteps. An honest and critical look at myself helped me to see that I don't have to believe every lying thought that comes into my head, whether it's from society or even from me. We are beautiful from head to toe, and even if it means reminding ourselves of this fact daily, so be it. This is not something you ever want to forget! You are beautiful!

These are life lessons that come with years of experience and acquired wisdom. I would experience hurt again in relationships, but it would never be completely devastating. During one of my toughest semesters in nursing school, I went through a horrible breakup. I was in my mid-twenties, and this guy I was dating was everything I ever wanted: looks, charm, education, ambition, you name it. I was busy caring for my son and studying for my classes, but I found the time to daydream about him constantly, writing his name in my study books like I was a teenager in love. But just one week before my final exam in the toughest subject, he broke up with me. I was frantic, maybe hysterical. My dreams of spending the rest of my life with this man as his wife was completely shattered. I can't explain how I read my textbooks through my raw, red eyes. How I pulled myself out of bed to dress and feed my son and even play with him. The sadness and depression were dragging me down into the deepest of depths. Not once did it occur to me to take a break from school or seek any kind of help. Somehow, I picked myself up, studied hard, and got the highest grade I'd ever gotten in nursing school. And, no, that wasn't the end of it for me. I still found the will to fall in love again, thankfully.

Relationships are important; they can help us build character and add to our overall health. But we cannot expect a relationship with another person to ultimately fulfill us or validate our existence. That's God's job! Losing or winning in love is just a part of life, I've learned. You enjoy people in all their complexities and imperfections. Keep the good, let go, and learn from the bad. When it's over, try to remember the good parts, the fun parts, and don't hold grudges. Learn to love yourself and forgive others through it.

I worry about young people, though, especially when I see statistics about the low rates of marriage and long-term relationships in the younger generation. It can be a beautiful thing when two people come together to build a life. Our communities would be much stronger with thriving, intact families raising the next generation.

I hope that we, as older women, are encouraging them to see themselves as beautiful the way they were made—in the image of the Creator who made everything beautiful in its own time. I hope we all learn that we are beautiful and deserving of love. It does not take a loving man to get you to discover that truth. All it takes is for you to look into the mirror with the right eyes and right frame of mind.

CHAPTER 10

Playing Nurse

A s a little girl, it was fun to run around Mommy's bar, eating snacks, staring at the grownups drinking, playing dominoes, and eavesdropping on their conversations. But as I got older, Mommy began to hover over me like a mother hen, and my visits to her place began to change.

"A bar is not the type of place for young girls to hang about," she would fret, watching over me as I hung around the adults.

Of course, I didn't agree, although I'm not sure Mommy really believed I was in any danger at her bar. All Garfield and I cared about was food and games! Mommy cooked us the most delicious dishes. Her famous brown stew and curried chicken, jerk and stew pork, stew beef, red snapper, fried fish, and rice and peas would bring in customers from across our town. We were kids just having a blast eating and hanging around adults. What was so wrong with that?

But it came to an end for me, and with my grandmother's grounding in the Anglican church and obsession with all things proper, I dared not put up a fight. I was what you would call a good girl, always wanting the approval of my teachers, grandparents, and my mother. Still do.

So I hung out less at the bar and more at Granny's. In addition to my five siblings, my grandmother took in renters from the villages who wanted to be near Kingston for the job and educational opportunities. Neighborhood kids were always coming by to play or to get meals, uniforms, schoolbooks, you name it. My grandmother kept her doors and her purse open for the entire community. She did it as naturally as waking up every morning. Later in life, when I would return to Jamaica in my thirties and forties, the house would still be filled with young people wanting to be around her, and she always had one or two picked out for me to help out with their financial needs—paying for textbooks, school uniforms. Trust me, saying no was not an option.

We were not rich, but we could afford things that were needed. My grandmother had hired help for cooking and help around the house, but we kids had a lot of chores as well. I half-heartedly watered plants and swept the veranda.

FIRST PATIENT

My grandmother, as I mentioned earlier, suffered from diabetes and hypertension for as long as I could remember. Caring for her was a family undertaking as ingrained into our routine responsibilities as sweeping up the yard or doing the dishes; every one of us kids was involved. Believe it or not, I enjoyed testing her blood sugar using a dipstick to test her urine. In those days, that was the only test available. (In her later years, I would travel to Jamaica to make sure she had the most advanced treatments and would treat her myself when I was on the island.) As a kid, I looked forward to giving Granny eyedrops to treat her glaucoma. It wasn't just that I got to play at being a nurse; I enjoyed caring for my grandmother in those intimate ways, feeling her breath on my face, touching her warm skin, brushing back her hair, and gaining the trust of a woman who I saw as larger than life.

As she grew sicker, Garfield or I would travel with her from May Pen to Kingston to see specialists for her multiple conditions. The trip to the big city was exciting in and of itself; Kingston was over an hour's drive from our home. Once we got into the city, I would immediately feel homesick; Kingston was intimidating and so crowded. And I couldn't wait to get through the visits and head back home.

The nurses I saw at Granny's doctor visits and in the public hospitals in Kingston never ceased to fascinate me. The two largest hospitals at the time were in Kingston and Spanish Town. Nurses in Jamaica were held in high regard back then and now. They walked the halls of the hospitals so confidently in their bright-white uniforms and starched nursing caps. They walked straight-backed and serious faced. Solid, serious women. I found it easy to trust them when they administered shots to me as a kid and when they took charge of my grandmother, leaving my brother and me to wait until they were finished. There was a competence, dignity, and kindness in these nurses that I could see myself achieving.

When I came to America, I only saw nurses from afar. Not many were visible in my area of the Bronx, although there were many nursing assistants. But not even that lack of visibility kept me from wanting to be a nurse as I worked at minimum-wage jobs. The profession had already been imprinted in my heart from a young age; I was going to be a nurse.

"If there's any angels in heaven, they're all nurses, male and female." President Biden said those words while he conferred the Medal of Freedom on me in July 2022. I admire our president, and I appreciate his respect for the nursing profession. But, alas, it wasn't an easy journey getting there.

CHAPTER 11

You Have to Run

T he late Christian pastor and writer Dr. Timothy Keller once said about life in New York City: You can have a great family life or a very successful career; you can't have both at the same time. I tend to agree. I wasn't a hedge funder or law firm partner, but I was working from sunup till sundown—for minimum wage. My mother and brother were still in Jamaica that first year, and my sister and cousin, whom I lived with, were hustling just as much. Those first years in America were a lonely, tiring existence.

Part of that was my choice. I know people who worked hard and played hard on the weekend, but I wasn't one of them. To me, the weekends were when I could pad my paycheck by making time and a half! Why would I waste that opportunity? Can I say something to my younger self? You needed to chill out!

The constant grind of hourly, minimum-wage work can isolate a person and narrow your focus to just one thing: work. But that was my life, making my hours so I could pay the bills and dreaming of making it to the next level. There were people who were living much different lives from me. I observed them hailing cabs from doorman buildings, dressed in suits and high heels, eating at fancy restaurants, and shopping at high-end stores. I was nowhere close to that life, nor did I expect to be at this point in my journey. I was keeping my head down and doing my thing, just trying to make it from day to day. Somewhere, deep down inside, though, I knew a better life was achievable. I just couldn't visualize it then.

I delivered the 2023 commencement address at the Frank G. Zarb School of Business at Hofstra University, where I got my MBA. I was so energized by the students' excitement at going out into the professional world. I, too, was fired up, recalling my experiences in business school, struggling with business and analytics and operations management, seeking help from my encouraging professors, and working with my student cohort. There I was, telling these bright students how they could overcome their challenges as they were heading out to high-paying jobs at top companies across the country. "Focus, determination, passion," were the words I wanted to leave with them. What a contrast to the challenges I faced in the 1990s as a low-wage worker with no upward mobility in sight. Sometimes, I did not think I could ever succeed. That commencement speech sure would have helped me back then! Thank God there were people in my life willing to encourage me and give me the tough love I needed to believe in myself and take the next step.

BIG BROTHER

When Garfield arrived in America, he was not impressed with my job at the grocery store. My slumped shoulders as I got ready for work every day told him all he needed to know.

"You need to push hard and go back to school." Garfield was not playing, and he would not accept my excuses. "How long you going to stay in that job?"

And as difficult as it was for me to consider making a change and giving up the security of my precious hours at my supermarket job, Garfield's presence and encouragement were what I needed to move on.

He was an inspiration. Garfield had already attended college and worked in banking in Jamaica before he emigrated to the US. He had a much easier time of it than I did as a new immigrant. Garfield, just eighteen months older than me, found a job as an accountant at a real estate firm in New York, a much higher-paying position with better prospects for advancement. That is why I will always stress the importance of education and its power to propel people forward. Despite facing discrimination in the workplace, my brother advanced professionally and financially because of his professional experience and college degree. But my lack of those things didn't mean that was the end of the road for me. No way.

Garfield likes to recite this old Jamaican saying: "If yu waan good, yu nose haffi run." You have to struggle if you want to achieve great things. New York required me to run and remain focused on my goals. So, for every opportunity that opened up, Garfield was there, telling me to reach for it.

A DAMASCUS MOMENT ON FORDHAM ROAD

One day, while walking home from a shift at the supermarket in the Bronx, I saw a sign for a nursing attendant school. It wasn't a flashy sign by any means, one of those places most people would hardly notice in a nondescript building way past its prime. But that sign stood out to me. I knew what a nursing attendant was, and it dawned on me that, hey, maybe this could be a stepping stone to what I really want. At the very least, it would give me an out from my miserable current situation. By that time, I was so demoralized and beaten down by that job that I was ready to take any job just so I wouldn't have to face those rude customers ever again.

So, I dragged my tired, pregnant self into the place. When they told me how much the course would cost—over $1,000—I nearly dropped to the floor in tears. My cashier job was just enough to pay the bills on the apartment I shared with my mom (I had moved out of my sister's place by that point). I had a baby on the way. The little I had left over in my paycheck let me have some fun every now and then. I had just gotten a microwave off layaway. I had paid ten dollars a week to the store until it was paid off. Whenever I heated up my food, I was never prouder to hear that all-paid-for DING! That feeling was almost as good as dropping off that last payment on a leather trench coat I'd had my eye on for months! That's how I was living; how could I afford to pay for a nursing attendant course? A little voice in my head said: "You'll pay for it the same way you paid for the microwave and the leather coat: little by little." So, I grit my teeth and went back to the supermarket the next day, and the next, and the next. I reminded myself: I was there for a purpose.

RUNNING AHEAD

As much as I hated that supermarket job, it gave me a perspective on life I'm grateful for to this day. My years in the Bronx among the poor and working-class equipped me with the best tools for surviving and thriving in America and finding the inner drive to accomplish my goals. I will always feel connected to the Bronx, to those folks on the BX12 bus heading to their second or third job, the street vendors, the recent immigrants taking ESL classes at storefront churches, the determined ones working day by day to climb out of poverty or just to be able to take their kids to the mall on the weekends.

It took that horrible supermarket job to help me build resilience and make me desperate for something better. I knew I couldn't stay there, that I was capable of more. Thank God for my brother for reminding me that I didn't have to stay, that even though nursing attendant school was expensive, it was not out of reach, and I was worth the investment. Were it not for education, I could not lift myself out of poverty, and I wouldn't be where I am today.

The pictures of my pinning ceremony show me grinning from ear to ear with my nursing school classmates, and that remains one of the happiest days of my life. I had graduated nursing school as a single mother, working full time as a nurse attendant, carless in New York City. On that December day in 1993, my entire family attended our intimate graduation ceremony—my aunt Azan (who stood in for my mother who had to attend a funeral back home), my son Kadeem, Garfield, and the nurses in my program whom I had gotten to know. I was valedictorian of the program, and although I have gained many degrees and honors since then, that associate degree in nursing from the Borough of Manhattan Community College was THE turning point in my life and is still deeply treasured in my heart.

CHAPTER 12

RN in the Flesh

T his full-fledged American missed Jamaica so much! The snow I had so looked forward to when I was in Jamaica did nothing for me now except trigger nostalgia for the Christmases in Jamaica when our grandparents would take us into Kingston to buy new curtains for the house and new clothes for Christmas service. Kingston came alive in December with people, music, and an air of excitement that the most beautiful white Christmas could not possibly come close to. I'll never forget hanging out the window on those drives to the city, daydreaming about what I would buy with my pocket money. Afterward, tired from shopping, we would stop at a restaurant before setting out again for the long drive back home. Garfield and I got tired of just talking about those days and existing on memories. Now, we make it a tradition to always spend the holidays in Jamaica from Christmas into the New Year.

In early 1994, just after graduating from the nursing program at Borough of Manhattan Community College, the reality of unemployment hit like a snowball to the face. There was no nursing shortage in those days, and most hospitals in New York City were not interested in nursing candidates with an associate degree. They wanted the students from New York University, Fordham, and the like. But that did not stop me from applying.

I went so far as to pay for a résumé service. And, boy, did that piece of bond paper look professional when they were done with it! I had a bunch of them printed, and my colleague and I did what few people would ever do for a job. We went, on foot, from hospital to hospital throughout the city, handing out our résumés to HR departments. It sort of worked. Some of the hiring people actually stopped to ask where we had gone to school before turning their backs on us. It was humbling and infuriating, but what was I going to do? Give up?

Months later, one of my clinical instructors from nursing school, Ms. Viola, who became one of my encouragers in chief, suggested I apply for an externship program, the Rita and Alex Hillman Scholars Program. It wasn't a permanent position, just a foot in the door, but I applied. Luckily, I was accepted and placed at Lenox Hill Hospital in the emergency room. To say I was grateful would be an understatement. I worked my butt off and tried my very best to impress every single nurse and manager I encountered by being a model employee: coming in early, offering to stay late, and having an upbeat attitude. I did all of that stuff, and it worked. It wasn't a dishonest ploy by any means; I really did want to make a great impression because this was my career, and I had finally squeezed my way into the door. The nurses were fantastic and supported me, and I could see from their example that I needed to get my bachelor's degree if I wanted to make this type of job my everyday reality.

THE GRITTY DETAILS

Before that externship at Lenox Hill, my first hospital job was as a nursing attendant, doing grunt work like bathing, toileting, and assisting them with their activities of daily living. I enjoyed it. The pay was more than twice what I made at the grocery store, and I felt proud that I was at least in my desired field. I could buy toys and clothes for my son, pay for a babysitter when Mom worked, and even have enough cash left over to brighten up our apartment. No more layaway microwaves!

As a nursing attendant in a busy hospital, you're critically necessary to patient care, and I know that now in a way I didn't back then. To any nursing assistants or attendants reading this, I hope you know how valuable you are to patients and other caregivers. Don't ever give in to the lie that you are the lowest on the totem pole.

Unfortunately, some of the nurses I worked with could be haughty and condescending. They looked down on the nursing attendants, never referring to us by name. If they wanted something done, they would yell, "Get the aide to do it!" That got on my nerves so badly! I vowed that once I became a nurse, I would never act that way.

I never reacted publicly to unfair treatment at work. I was a conflict avoider to the highest degree, and that trait tended to rub some people the wrong way. Speak up, they would say. Defend yourself and stand up to bullies! And I agree to an extent; it's the advice I'd give my own son. But at that age and stage of my life, I was still finding my voice and building my confidence. To me, those nurses and managers were in powerful positions. I had also grown up with a deep respect for authority figures; you simply did not talk back to adults or people in authority back in Clarendon. So, there were no showdowns or confrontations that I can remember, just me inwardly planning my exit and upward trajectory. I don't regret it, and I certainly do not apologize for my personality. People are different, and I have accepted over the years that we each respond to stress and conflict in different ways.

Instead of diving into conflict and confrontation, I chose to prioritize my mental health and plan for my future. These people would not always be over me, I told myself. I have always meditated and prayed, and those practices were vital when the mistreatment at work attacked my peace and joy. Plus, I had a loving and supportive environment at home: my mother, brother, and other family members helped me through my struggles by listening and encouraging me to stay the course. It's a blessing to be validated by people who genuinely know and love you. I knew I was not alone, and that helped me to quietly keep going.

The longer I remained in America, the more I learned that life would always bring challenges and that it was better to roll with the punches than to fight endless battles and wake up exhausted to fight another day. The fact is, I still had a ways to go in accomplishing my goal; I wanted to win the war.

REACHING BACK

A nurse named Doreen Wilson gave me the push I needed to finish my studies and finally get that bachelor's degree. Doreen, who passed away years ago, was approachable and friendly; she took the time to remember my name and talked to me about how she became a nurse. I loved working when she was on the floor. She spent hours with me, teaching me how to administer intramuscular and subcutaneous injections on an apple. Doreen was born in England, so she had a British accent. She was tall and curvy, had a beautiful dark complexion, and wore large-frame glasses over her beautiful dark-brown eyes. Doreen's bubbly personality lit up every room she was in. She was loved by her patients, the team she worked with, and everyone she came across.

We bonded as moms of toddlers. She had one daughter, Sasha, who was close in age to my son Kadeem. She would drive from New Jersey to the Bronx to pick up Kadeem and me in her Nissan Sentra. She loved Great Adventure and theme parks so much that she had an annual season pass. Some of the most fun we had was taking our kids to Great Adventure, even though I avoided the rides. But Doreen, in addition to being an excellent nurse, was just such fun to be around.

I had every good excuse in the world to carry on in my current role as a nursing attendant. Taking more classes would mean less time at my job, which paid my rent and bills. It would mean more time away from my baby. I was carrying a heavy load as a single mother, even though my son's dad was great and helped out as much as he could. Doreen gently encouraged me to think about it. Just think about it. I had a choice; I could stay where I was as a nursing attendant, or I could keep moving ahead, closer to my goal. It was a no-brainer.

RN, FINALLY

When the externship at Lenox Hill ended, it was back to reality. I was determined to get my bachelor's degree, but until then, I was still persona non grata at the big hospitals in New York. I went back to being a nursing attendant.

Then, one day, I received a phone call out of the blue from Lorraine Amorosi, a recruiter I had met at Lenox Hill. In her direct way, Lorraine got right to it. "Sandra, do you have a job yet?" The answer was a big, fat no. I was still sending out resumes and getting rejected left and right. I told Lorraine that no one wanted my associate degree. She replied: "Good, because I have a job for you."

Soon, I was back in familiar territory: the oncology department at Lenox Hill, but this time, I was full-time on staff, not an extern. When I entered the orientation, I realized how lucky I was because most of the nurses there were four-year degree nurses from NYU, and they wouldn't hesitate to let you know that. But I was confident with my associate degree, and I knew that wasn't the end for me. It was just what I could afford at the time. A lot of those nurses did not pass the orientation, or they left because the work was too hard.

Some advantages of the associate degree program were the practical aspects and the fact that we were drilled constantly on our skills. So, I had an advantage in being well-prepared to use my clinical skills. I did well in the three years I spent in that oncology unit. I made friends and bonded with a couple of preceptors (preceptors function as on-the-job nurse trainers, educators and leaders) who were also raising little boys. My preceptor, Michelle, was a fantastic nurse who taught me valuable lessons I still apply today.

The oncology unit was a tough place to work, as you might imagine. It was very busy, and the patients were very ill. This was all before the technology we have today, so there was a lot of manual work, like picking up and transcribing orders. Everything was on paper: charting, physician orders. But I enjoyed working there, minus the diagnosis of the patients.

I didn't know it then, but I was building a foundation that would keep me steady and ready during the COVID-19 crisis nearly thirty years into the future. In the oncology unit, I learned how to strategize to manage a heavy load of patients. In the unit, each nurse took care of eight patients. Nurses had to pick up their own orders from the physicians, which was no easy feat if the penmanship was not legible. We had to be extra careful of patient safety. The list of chemotherapy orders was long and confusing at times due to the sequence in which the medications needed to be administered. In addition to chemo, these patients often required blood and platelet transfusions, which come with their own set of strict guidelines for assessment, administration, and monitoring to detect complications.

Michelle, my preceptor and friend, was supportive as I learned all these new protocols. Our entire team—Dianne; Gina; Adrienne; Dawn, our assistant nurse manager; and the vivacious and fashionable Estelle, our receptionist—worked well together. I couldn't have asked for a better set of coworkers as a novice nurse.

We looked out for each other, making sure everyone was okay before we left for the day. Because of the care environment and the illness of our patients, we operated on a more personal level than in other care settings. It was easy to develop a relationship with the patients and their families and learn more about them. We grew so close to them that we knew who was coming on what day for what treatment, how many pillows they liked, and whether they liked fresh water or music playing in the background while they received chemo treatments. These details helped us to personalize their care, and those skills have helped me become a better nurse and leader throughout my career.

But as a young nurse and single mother, the emotional heaviness of the work took a toll on my mental health, and it soon became too much for me to carry. Around this time, my older brother was diagnosed with stomach cancer. I saw the difference in care given to patients in America compared to the care my brother received in Jamaica. Our cancer patients at Lenox Hill, for instance, had a variety of narcotic medications to choose from to ease their pain. However, when I visited my brother in Jamaica, we had to go to the pharmacy to purchase extra-strength Tylenol, which was prescribed by the physician. I watched as my brother cried out in pain, unable to obtain any relief from the care available in Jamaica as he faced his final days. It was difficult to go back to my job in the oncology unit after that experience. Playing back the memory of it is still very painful and is another reminder of how inequities in health care affect people around the world.

MAKING MOVES

There was an opening in the intensive care unit at Lenox Hill, and I went for it. My colleagues looked at me funny when I told them my plans. I explained my reasons for leaving, but they were still skeptical. The nurse manager for the ICU at the time was a legend. Everyone described her as tough, but I still went for the job, though it was a little scary going into the interview. She lived up to her reputation and was very stern through-out the interview, but I got the job anyway.

This was my first night job, and it couldn't have come at a better time. My son was in school then, so I could rest during the day. My mom dropped him off at school and cared for him in the evenings while I worked. That schedule fit my life for years, and it's another reason I love the nursing profession; the flexibility is unparalleled. I was able to earn advanced degrees, raise my son, travel when I wanted, and make a comfortable living doing all of that. I recommend nursing as a career choice to all young women and men I encounter. It is not easy to build a career or maintain a full-time job while raising a child. I am fortunate that my family was around me, willing and able to support me. I can't imagine what it would have been like if I had been on my own in New York as a single mom during those days. I have nothing but admiration and respect for the moms and dads who are doing this very difficult work today, raising a family while working.

CONTINUING EDUCATION

Throughout these job changes, I never stopped learning. After I graduated with my associate degree in 1994, I went on to St. Joseph's for my bachelor's degree. I took classes nights, weekends, anytime I wasn't working. I put aside money for the degree from my paycheck and used the $5,000 annual tuition reimbursement from my employer. It took willpower not to spend the money on other things! I did not have a car, so it was the Number 4 bus to the Number 2, and so on. It took me over an hour to get to school from the Bronx. I need to start thanking the New York City transit system for its important role in my education! Later, I received a master's degree from Leman College in 2010, and I took a break from school for a while.

When I finally had my dream job at Northwell, I was still taking advantage of tuition reimbursement benefits. I matriculated at the Frank G. Zarb School of Business at Hofstra (where I also received an honorary degree) and graduated with an MBA. This was one of the most difficult academic programs I have been a part of. But at the end of the program, I found out that wasn't the end of learning for me. One of my professors cornered me in at a pre-graduation event: Have you ever thought of going to get a doctorate? I thought about it. More school?! My son was an adult living on his own, so I had the time. I certainly had the interest. As my career matured, I had begun to compare and contrast the US health-care system with Jamaica's and was thinking of global inequities in health long before COVID-19 hit and gave me a platform to speak about these issues. I decided I would go for it. In 2021, I had my doctorate in health sciences with a concentration in global health and leadership and organizational behavior.

Why all of this education? Well, I felt like I was catching up. I was not a great student in high school and did not pass a lot of the courses I needed to get into college in Jamaica. I was still so lacking in confidence as a teenager; I didn't know the great things that were possible simply from my sweat and effort. It was only in America that I learned how to study and apply myself, and I loved it! Then, once my son came along, that propelled me even more. I was determined and adamant that I was going to give him the best, and that came through educating myself.

CHAPTER 13

Motherhood and Marriage

During this time of striving and climbing, my social life was terrible! I was always working, and my dreams were only getting bigger with every achievement. I was saving to buy a house and a car; my son was in a fantastic Catholic school (that was not cheap). I wanted a home because I wanted my son to have a yard to play in and to live in a community with good schools and extracurricular activities that would expand his life and development. I had enough intuition to know that the problems on the streets, the social neglect, crime, and poor schools could affect my son negatively if I stayed in the Bronx. Even though he was surrounded by positive male figures, like his father, Garfield, and other family members, I still worried. I wanted him to have just as full and wholesome childhood as I did, and I was willing to work hard, pulling several overtime shifts, to achieve that goal.

Family support was critical during those years when Kadeem was a toddler and a young boy. My sister, cousins, and I took turns babysitting each other's kids, and Mom would always step in when needed. People complain about the cost of childcare today, but I can't remember a time when babysitting was ever cheap. There is always a cost, and I had to take that into consideration. When I worked the night shift, it helped me save on babysitting costs because my mom was home. Then there was the trust element. My son would scream so hard when I left him at the babysitter—it would tear my heart out to leave him crying and so upset, but I had to work.

YOU'RE HERE AGAIN?!

Those overtime shifts did not go unnoticed. I was constantly at work, and it did not always go over well with my colleagues. Whether out of genuine concern or something else, other nurses would make comments: "You're here again?!" It felt like I was committing a crime by doing those extra shifts, even though I was only doing what I knew to create the life I wanted for my child. I grit my teeth through it. A few snide comments would not stop me from working despite the shame I felt. Soon, I started hiding at work. Yes. I hid in back rooms so that no one I knew would see me staying late or picking up an extra shift. Gosh, that made me so angry that I was made to feel ashamed for doing something honest, that I was working an honest living and yet people were being so mean about it.

SUBURBAN LIFE

The first home I purchased was in Rockland County. It was a beautiful house, a huge raised ranch with a big yard like I was accustomed to in Jamaica. The yard was perfect for my son to play and for us to host large, elegant parties. I made sure there was a separate dining room where we could sit at the dinner table and bond over healthy, home-cooked meals like my family did in Jamaica. I was set on reliving my childhood and bonding with my son, so we had one television in the family room and no TVs in the bedroom. On sunny days, we would eat outdoors on the extra-large deck. The community was quiet and tree-lined, with mani-cured lawns and lush gardens. I cultivated a beautiful garden that my gardener helped me to maintain. Finally, it seemed, I had the life I was meant to live.

After many years of living in the Bronx, the suburbs were a breath of fresh air—literally. It was just me and my son, as my mom decided to stay in the city near her friends and the convenience of public transportation. I can do this, I told myself after moving in. My son was in a great school, and the plan was to get him signed up for all the sports teams in the universe. Even before we moved to the suburbs, Kadeem had attended private Catholic schools and was a good student, so I had no doubt he could hold his own academically.

My daily commute to the city was long. I would be up in the dark before the sun came up and out the door to get to work. My days would be long twelve-hour shifts, and I would get home very late on those nights. It was exhausting. Although I had gotten what I wanted—the beautiful house in the suburbs—I was still in distress because I wasn't enjoying it. I hardly saw or spent time in my beautiful home. The idyllic suburban areas with the yards, beautiful trees and wide roads were only visible on my drives to and from the city. I couldn't get involved with the school PTA because I just didn't have the time. Worse, my son was now a latchkey kid going out to get the school bus and coming home to an empty house until I got home.

To make up for my absence, I would take my breaks around the time Kadeem came home from school so I could do homework with him on the phone. Those little phone sessions did so much for me; it was the brightest part of my day. I wished I could be home with him instead, though. By the time I got home late at night, we could catch up for a little bit. Then, it was off to bed to do it all over again the next morning. This dream life that I had finally achieved came with a hefty price tag. I had to constantly work overtime to pay for it. I was far away from my mom, family, and friends, who remained in the city. I had the comforts of suburbia, but I lacked community.

After a while, I began to resent this dream come true. My son was a teenager and very independent, so I was open to making another change.

At this point, around 2012, I had met my husband, and he could see that the long commute and time away from home were making me unhappy.

We decided to move. I sold the house, and we all moved back to the Bronx. I put my son back into a solid Catholic school, and we settled into a nicer area in a comfortable house as a family.

BACK IN THE CITY

But was I really ready to be back in the Bronx? No. Immediately, I wanted to get out. Crime was still rampant, and the streets and city life were still loud and chaotic. I was scared for my son because I was still working a lot and gone most of the day, leaving him on his own or in the care of family. During those days, home cameras were not as common, so I didn't have the ability to visually make sure he was home safe. Yes, he was in a good school, but he had to travel to and from school, and anything could happen. At least, that was my thinking—worry and anxiety every day.

I did sit him down on more than one occasion to explain to him as best I could the dangers he faced as a Black male in America. In his teenage years, we had the typical power struggles. I hated—absolutely *hated*—the way he dressed: baggy jeans and football shirts, whatever the kids in the city were wearing. I warned him that he would be judged harshly just for dressing that way. It fell on deaf ears.

"Why can't you just let me be a kid?!" he would complain, but I was afraid for him and how people would stereotype him. The thought of my son facing prejudice and mistreatment was sometimes unbearable, and my anxiety and fear made me a nagging mom at times, I admit.

I told him that if he should ever be stopped by police, he should comply to the best of his ability and be respectful and answer, "Yes, sir," or "No, sir." I didn't care whether that was the right or wrong way. I just wanted him to be safe.

God, I hated those conversations. I hated the fact that I had to have those conversations with him. This was not the way I had grown up. When I was in school, I came home to a house with an adult there, either my grandmother or her helper. There was a home-cooked hot meal on the table and all of that. There were no police or random bad guys looming as a potential threat. It bothered me that my son couldn't have that life.

RAISING SONS

Raising a young boy is not for the faint of heart. It might be controversial to write this, but I do think that a two-parent household is, in most cases, the best way to raise a child. Sons, especially, need their fathers. Kadeem had a good relationship with his father, but he did not live with us, so I absorbed the daily ups and downs of parenting—and Kadeem absorbed the impact of my ups and downs as well. I'm grateful that his father, my brother Garfield, and other family friends were good male influences in his life.

When he began to struggle with authority, I was at the end of my rope, although when I look back, I can laugh at some of our blowout fights. Once, his teacher called me at work and told me he was refusing to spell correctly. It's not that he didn't know how to spell the words; it's that he was REFUSING to spell out words. Instead, he would write his assignments using text shorthand like "txt" and "ppl" instead of "people." Mind you, he was a teenager! Oh, I was so steamed at this kid! You know how the rant goes. "I'm spending all this money for you to go to Catholic school, and this is what you do to repay me?! You can't even write out a word?!"

Thank God that was the worst of it. I never had to go to a police station, never had to go to the school for anything more serious than his little spelling vacation. And that's how I measured my success, which is unfortunate, but I think common for Black mothers. The worry and anxiety we feel for our boys are constant, and if we're single moms, it's so much worse. During the summer of 2020, in the aftermath of the George Floyd murder, I was overwhelmed with anxiety. I had been having the talk with Kadeem for years. I drummed it into him. "If the police stop you, put your hand on the wheel. Just keep your mouth shut, let them know when you're going to roll down the window," and so on.

"Just make sure I don't get a call that I have to come and identify your body," I would warn him. "Just comply."

I want to stress the importance of extended family and community in raising my son. And my hope for other moms is that they can maintain their ties to family and friends who are committed to helping them walk this parenting journey, which can sometimes feel like a gauntlet. My son has always been close to my mother, constantly chatting on the phone with her. And my brother always played a big role in his life. That extra layer of support eases the anxiety and worry for us moms. But it also gives our kids support; my son can talk to Garfield about things he won't talk to me about, and the same for my mom. It really does take a village, no matter how small. If you have one, treasure and nurture it.

LEAVING THE BRONX AGAIN

Over time, my husband and I decided to leave the Bronx. We bought a house and moved to New Rochelle, back to the big house, big yard, big trees life. My son was nearly an adult then and ready to be on his own. It was a time for change and growth. My marriage itself was struggling in more ways than one, and unfortunately, it ended within a few short years of that move.

My dream for my son was similar to what I dreamed for myself. I wanted him to have a great education, and I spent a lot of money making sure he went to the best schools to prepare him for a good college. These were the kinds of things my nursing friends and I commiserated about. When our kids were small, we dreamed out loud for them. Our long shifts, stubborn patients, arrogant doctors—they were all worth it because we were doing it so that our kids could someday grow up healthy, cared for, and hopefully follow the path we had laid out for them.

I had Kadeem's future all planned out in my head. As a tiny boy, he would immediately open every toy that came into his hands, take it apart, and put it back together again. My mom brain went to work overtime. Computer science! Engineering! Architecture! That's what he would study, I thought. I would buy him tons of VTech toys, trying to stir up the gift that I had envisioned would make him the person I wanted him to be.

But after high school and one year of college, he was done. "That life is not for me, Mom," he shrugged. He always liked fixing things and working with his hands and, most of all, just being independent. And that's how he has lived his life. He has been a successful electrician, and now he works as a mechanic with German car companies. He does his own thing on his own time and takes good care of his family.

I'm happy that he's happy and living his life the way he wants to live it. This son of mine has been a gift in every way, and I am proud that he chose his own way and not mine! Not only is he doing good work that companies pay him good money for, but he is also in a stable relationship and has a beautiful son.

Again, I am proud of my boy. He was the inspiration when I worked as a cashier and as a nursing attendant, when I was running to and from class between nursing shifts, and when I had my own big office at Northwell. I've always wanted him to be proud of me, and I wanted to give him a comfortable life in which he would want for absolutely nothing. I wish I had made zero mistakes in raising him, but I am so glad my imperfections did not harm him too much.

Right now, my aim is not to be a meddling grandma, which is always a temptation. I love my grandson, who is now three years old, and wish he could spend more time with me, although my busy schedule does not allow that. But I'm determined to allow my son and his partner to live their life on their own terms. I am there to help when they need me, but I respect their privacy. My son is very responsible, a good provider, and a dedicated father. I know I have nothing to worry about.

CHAPTER 14

Building Confidence
as a Leader

Marriage was bittersweet, I will say, without getting into much of the details. Even though it did not work for me, I continue to believe that a good marriage is a natural and the best foundation for a healthy family. It's not always achievable, but when it works, it can be a beautiful thing to witness and be a part of. Now that I'm in a healthy relationship, I can better appreciate the value of a healthy partnership that gives life to both people in the relationship.

Divorce is painful, even when you're the one who ended the marriage. The stress of the breakup can feel like death, it has been said. For me, it was a difficult time, another mountain that I had to climb.

One of the most difficult things about the divorce was dealing with the gossip at work. While I believe in being authentic and bringing one's whole self to work, I don't believe this authenticity involves telling all of one's personal business to coworkers. And some coworkers can be nosy! Too nosy! Some would ask outright what happened to my wedding ring. It was bad enough I was going through this terrible experience. I only wanted to focus on my work and not have to talk about my personal life. At one point, I even bought a different ring to deflect attention from the gap on my wedding ring finger. But some of my colleagues still noticed. Eventually, I just shrugged it all off and stopped answering questions in detail. This part of my personal life was for me and for the people I wanted to share it with and no one else. Can you tell this was a huge milestone in my personal development? I wish more women like me (nonconfrontational) would get there and learn to simply turn their backs on the gossipers and walk away with a smile. Just say no! No, ma'am. You don't get to demand from me the ins and outs of my life!

Today, I am in a relationship with someone I consider a true partner. He roots for me, champions my every move, and is down to travel and explore the world with me. The biblical concept of being equally yoked is so important to the success of a relationship. Being on the same page emotionally and spiritually, supporting one another, and not keeping score are great ingredients to start. Mine is a wonderful, life-giving relationship, which I highly treasure. As I shared earlier, there were times when I didn't think it was possible for me to have that kind of loving partnership, and that negative thinking began very early in my life. Thank God my thinking changed, freeing and enabling me to recognize and receive real love. It wasn't easy! Becoming the woman I am today took years of perseverance, patience, humility, and listening and learning from others.

CONFIDENCE AND COMPETENCE

Since the early 2000s, I have been obsessed with books by and about business leaders and their leadership philosophies. My brother Garfield thinks I'm crazy. He is quite happy not having the headaches of managing staff. But not me! I love giving back and sharing other people's professional journeys as they learn and climb. How did I even become this person, you may ask? I was never an extroverted, hard-charging type. However, through work, school, mentors, and reading a ton, I've learned that leadership skills can be learned and nurtured into excellence.

Anyone can be a leader—not just people with certain character traits. Some of the books that have influenced me the most are *The Mentor Leader: Secrets to Building People and Teams That Win Consistently* by Tony Dungy, *Good to Great: Why Some Companies Make the Leap and Others Don't* by Jim Collins, *Lincoln on Leadership: Executive Strategies for Tough Times* by Donald T. Phillips, and *The Contrarian's Guide to Leadership* by Steven Sample. Lastly, one of my favorite ways to relax is to read the *New York Times* "Corner Office" column.

In business school at Hofstra, case studies gave me a technical and practical view of problem-solving through teamwork and important lessons on how to lead effectively. Even when I may have the lowliest of titles and least experience on the team, I can still lead by example. Being excellent is not reserved only for people at the top. Insights from powerful and effective leaders have inspired me professionally and personally. These books dissolved internal fears and opened possibilities I previously saw as closed.

Long before business school, however, I was learning how to be a leader. Those skills were being honed when I practiced patience and self-control at my four-dollar-an-hour supermarket job; when I walked from hospital to hospital in the city handing out résumés, knowing the answer would be no; when I was shamed because I needed to work overtime to provide for my family; when I chose to see the beauty in myself and tune out the negative voices in society; when I mentor and encourage young people to stay in school and hold on to their aspirations.

When I tell a young nurse, "You can make it," I know of what I speak.

Now, no one can shame me for working too much (in their opinion) or wanting another degree. I learned through the stories and examples of other leaders that I have to walk the path laid out specifically for me to accomplish my goals: continually learning and pursuing my passion for improving access to equitable health care for all. Others are welcome to their opinions as they walk their paths, but those opinions have little to do with me or what I am doing. How I wish I had known that when I hid so others wouldn't see me working. I would tell them now: Thanks for your concern, but I'm doing what works for me!

Of course, I had many other lessons to learn along the way—for example, how to be humble and to seek advice from mentors who had walked the path before me. From Doreen, who was kind enough to slow down and show me the basics of nursing, to the tough nurse managers who led by example with uncompromising excellence, I had great teachers.

I learned to trust my own experiences and the fact that I had matured through them. So, yes, I did have a point of view that was worth listening to and worth sharing with others. Getting older and wiser also helped me get more comfortable in my skin; after a decade or two in New York hospitals, you begin to think you have seen it all.

Learning how to be a leader practically and intellectually also taught me that I have to be a realist. I had to make a spiritual contract with myself that I would not live a lie. Here was the deal: I wanted to climb beyond nursing at the clinical level to become an executive. That meant getting a high-quality education and putting in a lot of hours of work. That was the contract I signed with myself. I was ready to do the work, step by step, that would get me there. It wasn't a pipe dream; I saw other women like me doing it every day. I wasn't trying to become a ballerina or the Queen of England. I was confident that because I was already doing the work, getting good performance reviews, increasing my education, and growing more and more comfortable with being my authentic self, it was only a matter of time before everything would manifest in the flesh.

CHAPTER 15

Step by Step

Nursing can take you on a tour of the entire human body and intimately expose all the ways it can crack and break. In my twenties, after working in the oncology unit at Lenox Hill, I did a stint in the coronary care unit. I worked in that unit for about three years, building my clinical skills and strengthening relationships with my colleagues. Can I just say that being reasonable and agreeable goes a long way in any profession? People love to come to work when the environment is professional, people get along, and everyone is trying their best and gives grace to one another when they're having a bad day—or week or year! I have had challenging work environments, but they were few compared to the wonderful nurses, managers, and doctors I have worked with over the years.

Most of the senior roles I received came as a result of relationships with past bosses, colleagues, and longtime friends in the profession. I became an assistant nurse manager because my former boss was leaving her position and recommended me for her job. I was shocked when she called and told me what she planned to do. Me? An assistant nurse manager in the coronary care unit? Just a few years before, I could barely get a hospital to look at my résumé! She listed all the reasons she thought qualified me for this leadership role. She was naming qualities I had never even seen in myself. "You are emotionally balanced, bright, knowledgeable, clinically competent, patient, respectful, bring people together, charismatic, know how to teach, calm, and thoughtful."

I was flattered, but my mind began to race with doubt. Not only was I happy being a bedside nurse, but I was also good at it, and it gave me flexibility for childcare. I could schedule as much overtime as I needed. If I joined management, I would lose that flexibility and become a salaried worker—no more overtime. I could hear Garfield's voice in my head before I even asked his opinion: "But it would be a good investment in your future."

If you understand Jamaican culture, you will know that stability is very important. Very much like the basics of the American dream—a house, car, and two kids—Jamaicans prize having a good job with benefits that you can hold on to until you retire back to the island after all your decades of hard work overseas. You just can't walk away from a good, stable job! And that was what I had in hand. Still, I began to think about it and write down the pros and cons. Eventually, I went off my own script and took the job.

BECOMING ONE OF "THEM"

One of the big drawbacks of taking on a managerial role lay in my previous conceptions of nurse managers. As a staff nurse, it was common for my colleagues and me to view our managers as "they" or "them." We were the "we" or "us" who were working as hard as we could yet still felt misunderstood and taken for granted by "them," the managers. We were also in a union, which granted job security and protection.

So, there I was, skipping over my colleagues and leaving my union-protected job to join the dark side. To make matters worse, there was no formal interview process. One day, I came in to work and started my new job. The previous day, I'd been a nurse on the floor, just like my colleagues. What a mistake that was! The nursing staff, who had been my coworkers just one day ago, now eyed me with suspicion. I had become their manager with no advance warning.

"Why her? Why not someone else?" They questioned out loud and did not spare my feelings. They noted that I didn't have a master's degree and questioned my experience and ability to lead. Then, there were the implied accusations of betrayal: How could you cross over and become one of them?

Tension was thick in our unit those first couple of weeks. It was not fun for me. I carried my past insecurity wherever I went, unfortunately. There were several nights during that time when I would leave work in tears after a day of heavy-duty hazing. Some of the people I considered friends were the least supportive. But I was determined to show them not only that I could do the job but that I cared for them and our team.

It took a while—a few months—but the work environment began to change when they realized that I was a hands-on manager, right there with them every day. My nursing staff saw that I would and could do the work of patient care and leadership effectively and that I wasn't there simply to pull rank; we wanted the same things out of our work environment. I stayed in that role for three years.

ARE YOU SURE YOU WANT THIS JOB?

My next job was leading a challenging intensive care unit as a nurse manager. Even during the interview, the nurses warned me, "This is a difficult job. Are you sure you're up for it?" That particular unit had gone through several managers, had experienced high staff turnover, and morale was in the pits. This time, the hiring process was done correctly, and the staff had an opportunity to interview me. I made sure to zip my lips and reserve my recommendations on what I thought they needed. Instead, I listened. It paid off when I won the staff's respect early on.

The problems in that unit were not a secret. The staff let me know that they were tired of the turnover and the feeling that no one cared enough to stay in their unit. They felt neglected; they had needs that were going unaddressed. What did they want? Stability in a leader and someone who cared and could advocate for them.

It was hard work, and I hardly got any days off those first couple of years. But it was a crucible for leadership that added so much value, both for me and the staff. I went first for the low-hanging fruit, like making sure they had enough copy paper at their desk, that there were enough cables for the monitors, and that the cables were in a centralized location at the beginning and end of each shift. Those little changes meant less running around, less frenzy when a patient was being brought into the unit, fewer frayed nerves, and a happier staff.

It dawned on me that the unit simply lacked good processes to make the work more efficient and foolproof. The staff needed care and consideration. Just because they were caretakers didn't mean they didn't also need care. These good processes we developed together were quick little wins that made all our lives so much easier. Everybody benefited, especially me. I had a staff who trusted me and a unit that worked well.

WORKING WITH "THAT BOSS"

After a time, I plateaued out of that job and rose into other leadership roles. The hospital went through some major organizational changes. And eventually, I had a new boss. It was my turn to adjust. I don't want to be a hypocrite, and I certainly don't want to bash anyone. But here I was, leading a team of nurses in an intensive care unit and seeing good results, yet I was being led by someone who criticized me and did not appreciate or see my strengths.

My new boss was a challenge for me. Looking back, I can appreciate the value of this bump in my career. Everyone needs one—a situation or a person who causes you to stop and evaluate where you are, what you are doing, why you are doing it, and whether it is worth it.

I didn't feel that my new boss was fair in evaluating my work. His criticisms seemed more directed at me as a person than at my actual work. When I observed how he treated other team members, I could see the difference, and it felt personal to me, not professional. I could have been wrong, but my feelings are my feelings, and I'm old enough to know when to trust them. I became increasingly unhappy under his leadership.

There's nothing more demoralizing than having a boss whose goals are not aligned with yours. I told myself that by the end of 2015, I was going to resign from the hospital and start over fresh—a whole new career, new place, new everything. I began to look at houses in Atlanta. The houses seemed so big, and the grass seemed so green. I fantasized about leaving the New York winters behind for good. Maybe I would do something even bigger than move South, something more rewarding, like volunteer abroad.

Although the stability of work was always in the back of my mind, I was considering breaking free and taking a risk. Then, a recruiter reached out to me in December 2015 with a tantalizing proposition: a director role at Long Island Jewish Medical Center had just opened up.

The Northwell campus of LIJMC is enormous, taking up several blocks in the town of New Hyde Park. I had been in plenty of large hospitals, but this one was different. This position was more prominent than any of my other positions in more ways than one. LIJMC was an award-winning institution and well-known for its excellence in nursing care. The main building at LIJMC is an imposing, gleaming structure that, in some way, evoked capability and authority.

Dressed and ready for my interview, I looked up at the buildings and the impressive signage: Northwell Health, Katz Women's Hospital, Zuckerberg Pavilion. Was I intimidated? A thousand times, yes!

Previously, in my twenty-two years of nursing, every job I'd ever had was just a regular interview (except for that one with no interview). But for this role, there was a panel of at least a dozen people—nursing directors, executives, and physicians—when I entered the conference room. Talk about pressure. I sat at the head of the table and reminded myself that I had every right to be there. I answered all of their questions with full confidence that I was well suited for the role, and I felt very good at the end. Even when I walked into the building, it felt like a place I wanted to work; this new job was the one for me, I thought. But a week or two later, I heard from the recruiter that they decided to go with an internal candidate.

Worst Christmas ever! I felt so down. I was moping around again, thinking about moving to some far-flung country to work in an orphanage or start my own clinic. Again, it took my brother to talk some sense into me. It wasn't my ideal job, he reminded me. The role was director of medicine, and I was a critical care nurse. But I had fallen so deeply in love with the idea of myself as a director that I continued to grieve and mourn for this job that I never even had. Garfield couldn't understand why I was so upset. "You're a critical care nurse. You were just going to settle for this job. Why are you so upset?"

Maybe I had gotten too used to winning. Maybe, just maybe, I had forgotten all the years of rejection when I first graduated with my associate degree in hand and couldn't find a nursing job to save my life. Maybe I needed a reminder that sometimes, the answer is no—for now. That "no" does not mean you're incompetent, unqualified, or a bad person. It just wasn't the thing for now; it wasn't the end of me or the end of the world.

A few weeks later, I got a call from the recruiter asking if I was still interested in working for LIJMC. A director of critical care nursing post at the same hospital had just opened. Another panel interview later, and I was finally offered the job. I started in March 2016.

CHAPTER 16

Serving, Caring, Leading

For many years, part of my Sunday morning ritual was to go to Starbucks to sit at a communal table and read the *New York Times* "Corner Office" column in the business pages. The "Corner Office" column would feature interviews with CEOs from different companies and cover topics like what inspired them to be a leader and how they developed their leadership philosophy. On those Sundays in the mid-2010s, I was finally at a point in life where I could enjoy a day off and focus on my interests and hobbies. After over a decade of grueling hours and balancing a busy work life with motherhood and more, I could decide on a Sunday to plant zinnias or read the *New York Times* in my town's Starbucks. I learned so much from reading those interviews while I drank coffee and enjoyed the slow pace of a Sunday.

Taking the time to slow down and reflect and be grateful is good for the mind, body, and soul. On those lazy Sundays, I could allow myself to be truly thankful for my life and the people who helped me get from point A to point B, whether it was in my career, as a mother, or as a friend. For me, leadership is not simply leading an organization or a team. It's also leading by example. As a young nurse, I never could have imagined being an executive in a major health system, a national advocate for important health issues, and a mentor to many. But I had great role models, some of whom have been in my life for decades. Maxine Cenac-Carrington has been my professional cheerleader for years, helping me to build my confidence and pushing me to apply for the director role at Long Island Jewish Medical Center. Everyone needs a Maxine in their life. She noticed when I was being passed over and discredited by a former boss and pep-talked me into taking the leap to my next position. Maxine remains a constant cheerleader and a woman I truly admire.

THE ULTIMATE BOSS

One leader who has been a powerful inspiration is my current CEO at Northwell Health, Michael Dowling. You can read all about Michael's visionary leadership in his many books.[19] Even before the pandemic, Michael Dowling was an extraordinary leader who inspired many throughout the Northwell hospital system and beyond. When Michael speaks, you really feel like he's speaking to you. He speaks in a way that moves people to act—so much so that you feel like you could lift up Brooklyn Bridge when he's finished giving a speech. In his book, Dowling describes how the Northwell system, besieged by a lethal crisis, managed to treat patients and not be overwhelmed by the fast-spreading virus. He credits Northwell's size, its culture of preparedness that he said began long before he became CEO, and the courage and professionalism of health-care workers for the hospital's outstanding response. Although his leadership was critical during the pandemic, Dowling continually credits others for their contributions and shares successes with them.

Through difficult times like the COVID-19 pandemic and the protests of the summer of 2020, Dowling embodied great leadership. He spoke out against the injustice of the George Floyd murder and affirmed

---

[19]   Michael J. Dowling and Charles Kenney, *Leading Through a Pandemic: The Inside Story of Humanity, Innovation, and Lessons Learned During the COVID-19 Crisis*, Skyhorse Publishing, 2020.

his commitment to making sure that all employees at Northwell felt welcome by fostering an inclusive and supportive workplace. Dowling has taken public, courageous stances on gun violence, women's health, and, of course, the COVID-19 vaccines. He has been criticized by various groups, but not once have I observed him back down in the face of opposition.

It has been inspiring to watch and learn from him. I call him the ultimate boss because, despite his successes, he came from humble beginnings and has not forgotten his roots. His book *After the Roof Caved In: An Immigrant's Journey from Ireland to America* describes his beginnings in poverty and his immigrant journey in America. Dowling has had a long career in leadership and public service and an international reputation of excellence, but he easily connects with all sorts of people, a trait I've observed when he comes to our hospitals. People gravitate to him, even run toward him. Staffers at Northwell describe him as warm, inspiring, and a respectful leader who is visible, inspiring, respects and cares about people. Michael Dowling and leaders like him are the ones I look to as role models.

ADMIRING FROM AFAR

Another leader I admire is Indra Nooyi, the former CEO of PepsiCo. I have not met her in person, but I have followed her career, read her books, and listened to her talks. Nooyi has consistently been named among the most powerful women in the world. While at PepsiCo, she led the company in groundbreaking ways that facilitated growth and changed culture. Nooyi was also known for cultivating loyalty among the staff and her leadership team and taking a personal interest in their lives, even visiting some of their homes.

This getting into people's lives rang familiar to me. It's how my grandmother treated people around her, particularly those she hired to help around the house. She treated them as individuals, learning their names and unique family situations. Years after they had moved on to other things and places, they would come back to visit whenever they were in May Pen. They always appreciated and respected her for the way she treated them with dignity.

HEROES AT HOME

I also think back to my father, who never let circumstances limit his vision of what he could achieve. He showed so much courage as a political leader of our community—not stepping down even after being shot, threatened, and harassed for years by political enemies. He was a great community leader who cared about his constituents' lives despite their political affiliation. He had run many businesses over the years but later became distracted and lost oversight, causing the collapse of the businesses he had worked so hard to build. After he left Jamaica and moved to the United States, he worked a number of jobs to support his family. He never stopped working, although he had health problems that he ultimately succumbed to. My father took risks. He tried and failed, then tried and failed again. I am very proud of him for trying and for showing me the value of perseverance and tenacity.

My family role models helped me through the challenges of parenting and working and through my short marriage and painful divorce while I was a nurse manager in a busy critical care unit. Thank God for my family and their support through those rough times! They shared their networks and church families with me when I was too busy to build a community of my own. I am glad I never moved far away from them; in some ways, we were able to have our miniature version of May Pen right here in America. If it had not been for the leadership of my grandmother and my parents, I don't think I would have survived any of life's challenges.

Growing as a leader meant accepting all the struggles, heartbreak, exhaustion, joys, and triumphs of my past. The good and the bad both taught me valuable lessons. Because of the setbacks I experienced in my personal life, I'm quicker to give grace to a struggling employee; most times, I can honestly say, "I've been in your shoes."

When I think back to that weekend job in the Hamptons, I was so full of hope. I never expected the weekend to end with me being underpaid and cheated by that wealthy couple. I do my best now to treat people kindly and to empathize with and believe those who have had similar experiences. I may not always do this perfectly, but I do try and hope to get better at it. So many of us have experienced stereotyping, bias, hostility, and other forms of injustice. We need to be kind to one another because we never know what the person in front of us has experienced. The incident in the Hamptons occurred thirty years ago, but it remains a daily reality for so many people.

EVERY NAME, EVERY FACE

To this day, former colleagues are shocked when they run into me, and I remember their names. I make it a point to do that, and honestly, it's not hard for me. I prioritize addressing people by their names because when I was a nursing attendant, I remember being called "the aide" by nurses who refused to call me by name. I also remember that during COVID-19, when I couldn't see my colleagues' full faces through the masks, I wanted to have remembered something about them, even if only the color and shape of their eyes.

I had one of those encounters recently, running into someone I worked with decades ago. They had seen me on some television program, and we laughed together at the idea of me being a celebrity. "It doesn't matter how high you climb, you remain like one of us, and we really love and respect you for that," the person said.

Good leadership means looking people in the eye and being generally interested in who they are, what kind of day they are having, and how you can help them. So whether it's a transporter or a nurse having a rough day, I want to be able to call them by name and let them know they are seen. It's what I would want for myself from my leaders.

Part III

THE COVID-19 PANDEMIC

CHAPTER 17

The Longest Wave

I n April 2023, I flew to South Carolina to participate in a program
with several health-care professionals at the Medical University of
South Carolina. The panel was convened to discuss what would
come next now that COVID-19 was no longer deemed a health emergency. It was a lively discussion on what we had seen during the crisis as
health care providers and the lessons learned, among other topics.

First, there was the reality check that COVID-19 remained a major
cause of death in the United States. By mid-May 2023, the *New York
Times* was reporting that COVID-19 was still claiming over a thousand
lives per week and had killed over a million people since 2020.[20] People
were still being infected and the rate of vaccinations had slowed precip-
itously. It's like we chose to be done with COVID-19, but COVID-19
was not done with us.

---

[20]   Lazaro Gamio, Eleanor Lutz, and Albert Sun, "As Emergency Ends, A Look at
Covid's U.S. Death Toll," *New York Times*, May 11, 2023, https://www.nytimes.com/
interactive/2023/05/11/us/covid-deaths-us.html.

To make matters worse, the problems in our health-care system exposed by the pandemic—health disparities and inequality, the politicization of public health, rising social problems like gun violence and deaths of despair—were not getting the attention they deserved. The media debates were less focused on people than in 2020. Politics, the economy, inflation, and interest rates were the hot topics. The fire to solve injustice and inequity was running low, reconciliation fatigue was setting in, and promises and programs were beginning to lose support and funding.

STILL NOT BACK TO NORMAL

From where I stand, however, COVID-19 remains a major societal threat, just in a different way than we experienced in 2020–2021. As one of my colleagues put it, "This [aftermath] may be the longest wave of COVID-19." And by saying that, I am not minimizing the suffering and the tragic losses of the first wave in 2020. Not at all. But the sheer number of people who continue to suffer and will continue to suffer in the years ahead cannot be ignored.

Long-term COVID-19 and its effects have put people out of work, on disability, and living vastly different lives than before their infection. Some children have lost one or both parents to the virus. Some families have lost loved ones. People have lost businesses and jobs. And many will never fully recover in one way or another from the stress and anxiety of the pandemic.

The Facebook group Young Widows and Widowers of Covid-19 had over a thousand members at one point, sharing their struggles of losing a loved one to the virus. *The Washington Post*[21] recognized the group and others like it as a haven for grieving people who needed validation and support when the rest of the country was clamoring for a return to

---

[21] Tara Bahrampour, "For Those Who Lost Loved Ones to Covid, There Is No Return to Normal," *Washington Post*, June 8, 2021, https://www.washingtonpost.com/local/social-issues/covid-widows-reopening/2021/06/07/7a55f9e6-c3bc-11eb-8c18-fd53a628b992_story.html.

normal. For these widows and widowers, their lives would never be the same. Neither would the lives of the small business owners who closed up shop and never reopened, the people who lost their jobs and could not find another one, and the ones who continue to struggle with the psychological effects of the fear and isolation brought by the pandemic. We are still learning about the effects of education loss among children and the social effects of school closings. Many people feel they are simply existing, while others feel they might want to stop existing because of having lived through COVID-19.

PLANS TO ADDRESS INEQUITY
ON THE CHOPPING BLOCK

Even before the pandemic, Northwell and other health-care organizations were actively battling health disparities in innovative and effective ways. For instance, we had begun a program that used artificial intelligence to address the problems of maternal mortality. But since the end of the COVID-19 emergency, that and similar programs have faced steep budget cuts. Luckily, Northwell's Maternal Outcomes Program showed some promising preliminary results, and has received funding for further research. Some hospitals, appreciative of their staff's valiant efforts and sacrifices during the pandemic, signed labor contracts with huge pay increases for nurses that were certainly well deserved. However, some hospitals are now unable to afford these pay raises. What does that mean for the hospitals? Some may go out of business, merge, or make staff and other cutbacks in areas where vulnerable people need care the most.

Then there's the politics. During the early days of the pandemic, the entire country rallied around health-care workers, and it was a wonderful feeling to be supported as we worked during those terrifying shifts of spring 2020. Although I never took advantage of it, it was nice to be given preference in the grocery store line if you were wearing scrubs in 2020 or to have someone say, "Thank you" or "I appreciate you." Those days are over!

Politicians and company executives gave lip service to the importance of programs addressing nursing burnout, diversity, and equity and increasing opportunities for advancement, recruiting, and retention. But in the last couple of years, as the political conversation grew more and more heated, I witnessed my nurses getting abused, physically and verbally. Patients were lashing out, bringing their conspiracy theories with them, and expressing frustration and anger by targeting health-care workers.

COVID-19 has not left us, I don't think. In these next few chapters, I will describe my experience, from the first wave to the omicron variant. I won't lie to you. It is difficult to even think about some of the terrible scenes I witnessed in the critical care unit from mid-March 2020 through the end of 2021. I do want to highlight how our team of leaders and nurses worked so hard for our patients and how we used all our professional, clinical, leadership, and organizational skills to provide the best care possible. I am so proud of that and everyone I worked with during those months.

There are plenty of fantastic books by medical, research, and political experts that offer a broader perspective on the pandemic. This book is not that. What you will find in these pages, however, are my experiences and my perspective. For a comprehensive and excellent account of the Northwell Hospital system's planning and response to the COVID-19 crisis, you can read our CEO Michael Dowling's book, *Leading Through a Pandemic: The Inside Story of Humanity, Innovation, and Lessons Learned During the COVID-19 Crisis.*

CHAPTER 18

Ringing in 2020

I ended the 2019 holiday season full of joy and hope, with the highest of expectations for the year 2020. I love going home to Jamaica at the end of every year, something I have done almost annually for the last twenty years. The holidays give me time to reflect on the past year and to think about what changes I can make in the new year. It's not about resolutions; I take it a lot more seriously than that. For me, every new year represents a rebirth, a restart, a refresh. And being home in Jamaica is the perfect place for that to happen.

My late friend Colin Hylton had invited Garfield, some friends, and myself to a party in an affluent neighborhood in Kingston that I had been anticipating for some time. Whether it's weddings, high school reunions, or other social events, I love getting dressed up in something sparkly and dancing the night away with friends and family, especially in Jamaica. It's always a joy to celebrate the life I have been given and the person I have become after many years of study and work. And I had plenty of things to celebrate that New Year's Eve. I was in a wonderfully challenging executive role at Northwell, my family was doing well, I was close to finishing my doctorate, and I felt and looked great. There was good reason to dance and raise a glass or two to 2019 and to what lay ahead in 2020.

We had a fabulous time. Kingston was colorfully sizzling with holiday excitement and visitors from abroad. The outdoor party venue sparkled with decorations and colorful stringed lights of red, blue, gold, green, you name it. Everyone was dressed to the nines—gowns for the ladies and island formal for the men. There was an artist creating an ice sculpture of the figure 2020; the sculpture was larger than life, maybe the size of a mid-size SUV. I watched as he carefully chiseled and sculpted the numbers under the sparkling lights of the party and starry skies. At one point, he stepped back to observe his creation, and I couldn't take my eyes away. This guy was so meticulous about his work! He went back to work sculpting slowly, making it close to perfect even though it would exist only for that one night. That's what I wanted, too: a perfect night to hold in time to kick off a perfect year.

The sculptor finished right about one minute before midnight, just in time for the large, beautiful sculpture to be unveiled as we cheered and brought in the new year. As the fireworks popped and color exploded in the night sky, I said to myself, "What an absolutely perfect night." I was among people I loved. I was nicely dressed. And I thought, "Wow, this is going to be a wonderful year."

DANGER AHEAD

Unlike some of my friends who avoid the news (too much bad, not enough good), I like to keep abreast of what's happening. I started hearing about the coronavirus in China in December 2019. I was in school at the time, and my doctorate concentration is in global health, so I had more than a superficial interest in this mysterious virus that was causing trouble in Wuhan, a place I'd never heard of before. In addition, when I got back to work from Jamaica, one of my doctors began ringing the alarm about a new virus that may be spreading from bats or pangolins to humans: "Sandra, I'm talking to my friends in China," she said, "and this is not gonna be good."

Indeed, in December 2019, intelligence officials from the US and other countries were well aware of a Chinese media report about the outbreak of coronavirus cases in China, and the Wuhan Municipal Health Commission, in a public statement on the outbreak, said it had identified twenty-seven cases.[22] Of course, none of these government-level discussions were in the public conversation at the time. It was only as the media reports began to increase coverage that the US public began to take notice. But even when the first US case was found in Washington State, most people probably never expected what was coming in just a few weeks.

COVID-19 reminded us that the world is smaller than we think. When people move around, so do viruses, diseases, and everything wanted and unwanted. So, as my doctor friend described the rates of infection in China in early January, I figured the virus would eventually find its way here.

What I didn't know was the impact it would have on the United States and the world. I thought that, given our advancement over the years, we would have learned how to deal with contagious viruses and contain them as we had done with Ebola or other viruses and diseases. It was sad to hear of people dying in other places, but I never thought we'd ever see that here in America.

At that time, I was director of patient care services for the critical care division at LIJMC, about four years into my tenure at Northwell Health. My job was to manage the clinical and other operations of the division, ensuring safety, regulatory compliance, teamwork, and camaraderie among the team of nurses, patient care technicians, unit receptionists, and other patient support teams.

My doctor friend, an intensivist in the cardiothoracic ICU, was advising the nursing staff to wear masks and not touch their faces. I

---

[22] "COVID-19 and China: A Chronology of Events (December 2019-January 2020)," Congressional Research Service, May 13, 2020, https://crsreports.congress.gov/product/pdf/r/r46354.

followed that lead, and the staff was beginning to take those precautions as well. This was in late January to early February 2020, when many hospitals were not yet requiring masks. At Northwell, we had a plentiful supply of masks, gowns, and boots, and throughout the crisis, we would never run out of PPE.

My doctor friend grew more and more concerned as news spread of infections in Washington State, Chicago, and California; these were mild cases of people who had traveled back to the US from China, but the news was still chilling for some of us health-care workers. We remembered the scares of SARS, MERS, and Ebola outbreaks of the 2000s and 2010s; we didn't want to have to deal with those protocols again. To make matters worse, the political atmosphere was growing more and more charged over limiting or blocking entry to the US and quarantining international visitors.

My doctor friend was even more serious now that the virus had reached the US. While I listened to her, I remained calm because it's not my personality to get flustered about things. My strategy was to collect information, assess the problem, and then make a plan. While I could see the worry in this doctor's face, I wasn't anxious. Not yet. I decided to watch the news and wait for guidance from my organization. In the meantime, I took my friend's advice: I always wore a mask and washed my hands like crazy.

THE FIRST PATIENT

On March 7, 2020, the first COVID-19 patient came to the ICU at LIJMC. He was a white male in his fifties. At this point, there was no denying the virus was wreaking havoc in other countries and was pretty much knocking on our doors. Reports of strict lockdowns and skyrocketing infection rates were emerging from Italy. In the coming weeks, the pictures of the devastating deaths in Bergamo, Italy, would be widely broadcast, striking fear across the globe. The stories from China and Italy were chilling warnings for hospital systems across the world.

When that first ICU patient arrived, other hospitals in the Northwell system were already treating and admitting COVID-19 patients. There was no test to administer to patients who presented to the emergency rooms. They would be asked a series of questions, including whether they had traveled overseas, and their symptoms (temperature, fatigue, body pain, difficulty breathing, and so on) would be assessed. Many patients who were young enough or had mild symptoms could be sent home to manage the illness. The very sick were admitted based on criteria (respiratory distress, blood oxygen levels, for instance) determined by Northwell's clinical advisory team.[23]

At this early point in the crisis, all the infectious disease personnel, physicians, and nurses in our hospital were involved in caring for this very sick individual, strategizing to provide guidance to the nursing staff on treatment and how to avoid cross-contamination. This amount of attention and staff directed toward this one ICU patient would not last for very long, unfortunately. Within a week, the Northwell network of hospitals had admitted hundreds of COVID-19 patients, and staffing became a serious challenge.

I felt confident that hospital leadership, meaning LIJMC and Northwell Health System as an organization, was committing all resources to the crisis and that the Northwell system was ahead of many other health-care systems in its COVID-19 strategy. Our top leadership was present and visible. Communication from the top was frequent and transparent. Of course, the nursing staff was concerned and had lots of questions, but everyone was ready to begin the work.

As the director of the ICU units at LIJMC, I would need to provide one-to-one care for

this ICU patient. To protect the nurse assigned to him and other patients and staff from infection, we also added a patient care associate (PCA) to ensure that anyone entering the room had PPE (booties,

---

[23] Northwell's clinical advisory team was a component of the system's incident command structure. The clinical advisory team, led by Northwell's top physicians, had various capabilities and issued alerts, policies, best practice guidelines, and clarifications on clinical policy.

goggles, gown, face mask, and gloves). All entrants to his room needed to be completely covered and then appropriately disrobed upon exit, performing proper hand hygiene throughout.

That system worked for a couple of days. Then, the volume of patients ticked way up, as did the severity of their COVID-19 symptoms. At first, the patients did not require the ICU. They would come into the hospital and be admitted to a lower level of care. Soon, many would take a turn for the worse with deteriorating conditions. It was frightening the quick rate at which patients would seem fine, then, in a matter of a few hours or overnight—or sometimes even minutes—would begin to struggle for breath and fail, or "crash," as the doctors called it.

Northwell's clinical advisory team was working hard behind the scenes to develop protocols and guidelines for the staff on how to treat patients, and these policies would be communicated to frontline workers. While the sickness of the patients was overwhelming, we knew that our top minds were at work on the best ways to treat them.

Still, our stress levels and fear of being infected did not go away. How could they? The nurses on my team were young, middle-aged, with families of their own. Some had elderly parents or families with existing conditions. I also want to stress that some of our nurses were new to the profession and recently out of school. These young nurses in their twenties and thirties were scared, no doubt, but courageously showed up to work every day during the biggest health crisis of our lifetimes. Hundreds of patients were coming to us on a daily basis. Our hospital typically has forty-eight ICU beds scattered across the medical, surgical, cardiothoracic, and coronary units. We were about to find out that this wasn't nearly enough.

FRIDAY THE 13TH

On the afternoon of Friday, March 13, I called my team to a conference room. As you can imagine, they were not very happy about this surprise meeting on a Friday at 3 p.m. We had long planned our weeks so that by noon, we could all start easing into the weekend. It was our way of establishing some work-life balance, and we had come to depend on that schedule. But that day, once they all sat in the conference room, I broke the news I had been given. "We're gonna have to open another ICU space. Now."

My bosses had designated a unit that had been out of use to be retrofitted to accommodate twelve additional ICU beds. This was on the sixth floor of the main building, where you can now find a six-bed extension of the medical ICU. This was an older part of the hospital that still lacked some of the more modern amenities, including individual private rooms. This was an older part of the hospital that still lacked some of the more modern amenities, including glass walls and newer floors. While some of the wiring and infrastructure existed for monitors, there were no actual monitors in the space. The job was to resurrect the space by redoing the wiring, installing monitors, and making sure everything was safe and ready for patients that very Friday night.

Faces drooped at the table, but we had no choice. I said to one of my managers, "Let's walk up to the space. Maybe seeing the area would help them feel invested in the project."

Construction workers were there when we arrived, pulling wires, raising hell with drills and whatnot, and everything was covered in dust. The space didn't look anywhere near ready. "What time do you think we're gonna be finished?" I asked the contractor.

"I have no idea," he replied. "We still have a lot of work to do."

I talked to the bioengineering guys, and they said the same thing.

I reached out to my boss. "I don't think this is gonna be ready for tonight. We've been here all day, exhausted," I said. "I think the best plan is for us to go home and come back in the morning and open up this new unit." Thankfully, she saw things my way. We both could agree that it would not be safe to move critically ill patients at night in any case.

Our non-COVID-19 surgical critical care unit patients would be placed in this redone unit so we could free up existing private rooms to accommodate critically ill COVID-19 patients. We chose this particular population of non-COVID-19 patients because the census and severity of illness were lower compared to patients in other critical care units.

Every move was strategically considered to prevent patient harm while meeting the needs of the wave of COVID-19 patients coming at us.

This refurbished unit would be more of an open area. At that time, COVID-19 patients each had their own rooms with locked doors, completely contained. Once we moved those non-COVID-19 patients to this open area, we would have thirteen beds with private rooms in the surgical ICU for the COVID-19 patients.

We pulled it off. That Saturday morning, our team of leaders, staff nurses, and patient care technicians who volunteered to come in went to work moving the patients and setting up this new unit. Luckily for us, the acuity in the surgical ICU patients was low, meaning the patients were not very sick, so the task was not too risky.

A few hours of backbreaking work later, it was done. We got the patients settled in the new space, did a debrief at the end just to make sure everybody was comfortable with how we were leaving things, got everyone to sign off, and we were good to go. I typically ensured my leadership team did their morning huddles and end-of-day debriefs; these huddles informed our strategy going into each day. Part of the strategy was also reviewing our previous decisions and actions, looking to repeat our successes and learn from our failures.

I went home that Saturday feeling like we had accomplished something really great. On Sunday, I did a quick check-in to make sure the unit was operating okay. I spent the remainder of the weekend working on my doctoral research, confident that I had probably helped solve the biggest problem I would ever have to face with COVID-19.

But on Monday, March 16, when I returned to work, it was an entirely different scene. The ICUs and the other units were unrecognizable from how we had left them on Saturday. It was as if a tsunami had passed through the hospital.

CHAPTER 19

The First Wave

E very bed in the traditional ICU was occupied, and every private room was filled. COVID-19 patients were everywhere you looked. The entire hospital was a war zone. We walked into the units in full gear, covered from head to toe as if armed for battle. It was a completely different place from the way we'd left it. Isolation signs were slapped on doors. Direct care staff were dressed in personal protective equipment from head to toe, with face shields masking their grim expressions. But you could see the fears and the tears in their eyes as they ran around all day, just running from patient to patient. Overhead, the PA system made announcement after announcement in quick succession, like an auction: Cardiac arrest. Respiratory arrest. Rapid response. Fifth floor, sixth floor, ninth floor. All day, it continued nonstop.

Over the span of just two days, one weekend in March, our lives transformed. That Monday, my business suit and heels came off, and I was in scrubs and clogs for the next two and a half years.

From Monday, March 16, 2020, it was nonstop: long, hard days that stretched into the night. Our hospital, like others in the New York metro area, was being heavily hit with patients. The systemwide peak in those early days was 3,425 COVID-19 patients on April 7 plus over 1,500 non-COVID-19 patients on that same day.[24] There were so many aspects of administrative, management, and clinical care to deal with this onslaught of sick patients: where to put them, how to care for them, who would care for them, and so on. Decisions were being made quickly at the institutional level, and each unit below had to be laser-focused on executing their tasks to the highest degree of professionalism.

HOW MANY CAN YOU TAKE TODAY?

Before COVID-19, a typical day for me involved huddling with my team to plan for the day; reviewing operations, expected patient admissions, surgical volumes, and where the patients would be placed; and putting out unexpected fires—that sort of thing. I also participated in patient rounding, staffing, and a lot of meetings, probably too many meetings.

When COVID-19 arrived, in some ways, my days became more streamlined. From the top-level Northwell executives to the intake specialists, everyone had a single focus, and all our guns were trained on a single enemy. Other patients were still being treated—cancer and other critically ill patients, for instance—but there were few other distractions once the COVID-19 surge began.

All my strategic thinking, management skills, and creativity went toward my particular area of the COVID-19 fight, whether it was filling staffing needs or moving patients in and out of critical care units. We would receive a directive from the top, and it would be my job to ask the questions. "Let's look at our facility, and if this surge happens, where are we gonna move first? Where are we gonna open ICUs?" Our team would assess the space available, do risk assessments, and come up with a plan that we would then execute.

---

[24]   Michael J. Dowling and Charles Kenney, *Leading Through a Pandemic: The Inside Story of Humanity, Innovation, and Lessons Learned During the COVID-19 Crisis*, Skyhorse Publishing, 2020, Chapter One. Chart: Inpatient Census: Covid-19 vs Non-Covid.

LIJMC is located in New Hyde Park and is probably the largest tertiary care institution there, although there are several smaller community hospitals around us in the Queens area. You may have read the media reports of public hospitals struggling with heavy caseloads and low quantities of PPE and supplies in March and April 2020. Well, one of the advantages of being a large, integrated hospital system is the ability to share resources and support smaller institutions. Every day, no matter the volume of patients, I would have to answer the request: How many patients can you take today? Some days, I may have had the beds but not the people to staff, or vice versa. However, my staff will tell you that no matter how tight our bed or staffing situation, "Sandra is gonna say yes."

And they were right. My philosophy was we can't ever say no. We just have to find the yes. As much as we were hurting, a community hospital didn't have the capability to care for these very sick COVID-19 patients nor the capacity to build out the way we did. After a while, the nursing staff stopped asking me and automatically tried to find a yes for every bed request. Everyone was on board with helping our community hospitals that simply couldn't manage the volume flooding into their emergency departments.

In addition to patients coming through the emergency department, we had ambulances dropping off patients to our ICUs from within the Northwell health system in a practice we called load balancing, which kept a single institution from being overwhelmed with patients. The staff didn't always appreciate the practice, and we had to explain it to them. They would say, "We're already being slammed. Why can't these patients stay at Forest Hills?" But load balancing saved lives, as our CEO described in his book. Over seven hundred patients were transferred from two of our most overwhelmed hospitals in Forest Hills and Valley Stream between March 16, 2020, and April 24, 2020, and over a four-week period, 423 critically ill from Forest Hills and 278 from Valley Stream were moved to other hospitals.[25]

---

25   Michael J. Dowling and Charles Kenney, *Leading Through a Pandemic: The Inside Story of Humanity, Innovation, and Lessons Learned During the COVID-19 Crisis*, Skyhorse Publishing, 2020, p. 10, Chart, Load Balancing; p. 12.

FEAR AND EXHAUSTION

My phone was always on. Every day, at home and at work, there was never an off moment. As a leader, I was expected to make critical decisions and answer the questions my nurse managers did not feel comfortable answering themselves. Some days, I don't know how I made it home. I was so exhausted from the sixteen-hour shifts. Stairwell B in the main building became a refuge for me, where I could just lean on the railings for two to three minutes, close my eyes, and breathe. Then, it would be back to the floor again to deal with whatever crisis was occurring.

Falling into bed was a relief. Somewhat. My house felt cavernous when I arrived home some nights. I felt a deep sense of aloneness, not having anyone to talk to about what I was experiencing at work. The aloneness felt worse once the lockdowns went into full effect, and the people that I cared for and loved were hunkered down in their homes or working at the hospital, putting themselves in danger of infection.

Prior to COVID-19, I never liked FaceTime. But during COVID-19, it became my best friend because that's how I connected with people on the "outside." Friends and family were concerned for me and other hospital staff. How were we coping? How were we protecting ourselves? The answer: Taking it day by day.

I tried hard not to think about my fear of infection because I wanted to be courageous for my staff, but we were all terrified, and each day we showed up to work, we worried that day was our turn. A few nurses had gotten the virus, and we lost a few staff members across the system, so we knew our vulnerability. Those of us with elderly or sick family members were even more scared and had voluntarily cut ourselves off from our family so we wouldn't endanger them. Still, most of us kept showing up to work every day.

Personally, going to work helped me deal with the anxiety, worry, and isolation. At work, I was doing something worthwhile with hundreds of other committed people. There was a strong sense of solidarity among the staff, and I still feel it today when I visit. We hug each other tightly and for a long time because we remember what we experienced together, and it's a bond that will never go away. Back in 2020, I would have felt even more helpless if I had decided to sit at home and wait out the emergency. I wanted COVID-19 to come to an end, and I felt that the more hands were on deck, the sooner COVID-19 would disappear.

On March 11, 2020, the World Health Organization declared that COVID-19 was a global pandemic. All hospitals were ordered to stop surgical procedures except for emergencies. That meant that all of our operating rooms were shut down. We suddenly had the post-anesthesia care unit, or PACU, and the ambulatory units that had monitors at our disposal. Every inch of suitable space was conscripted for ICU use.

The additional thirteen-bed unit we'd built on the sixth floor was useful but not nearly enough to cover the volume of patients streaming in from emergency care. Across LIJMC, dozens of beds were being added daily to accommodate the patient surge. I imagined it was the same across the Northwell system. Until May 2020, when the peak ebbed, the main question on everyone's mind was: Where do we place these patients and maintain safety for them and the staff?

THE TRAVELERS

There were more questions. Like, who's going to take care of these hundreds of patients? How do we staff these new units? In came the traveling nurses. The pandemic emergency mercifully resulted in relaxed regulatory requirements, allowing out-of-state nurses to work in New York without a state license. They arrived from the West Coast, the Midwest, the South, and all across America. These people had seen the news reports about inundated New York hospitals and felt compelled to help. We were glad for their enthusiasm and their courageous spirit.

Even before the traveling nurses arrived, we started with overtime every day, cajoling nurses and other staff to come in on their off days and stay late, offering them all kinds of deals. Just come in, we would say. "If you can't come at eight, then come at ten, come at twelve. It's okay." We had to reimagine the work assignments, coming up with creative ways to use the staff for patient care. We were like machines, humming, working all the time, brains thinking ahead, feet rushing to patients, hands washing, washing, washing. There was no time to stop and think. We just kept moving.

The traveling nurses were more than welcome, but they presented their own challenges. First, there wasn't enough time to assess their competency. I had to make judgments based on a résumé or scant bio that listed where this person worked in the past, their specialties, and the things they had done. There was no time to call references. Luckily, our incredibly intelligent educators at LIJMC worked very hard to onboard them and orient them to our systems and hospitals so that we could maintain safety standards. And once they made it onto the floor, we could give them more training.

The other pool of people who helped the critical care staff were the operating room nurses and ambulatory surgery unit nurses. While their skills and specialties are different from the critical care pool, these nurses stepped up in a huge way and were a great help. Again, because of the emergency orders in place across the country, the governor of New York temporarily suspended certain laws and regulations regarding licensing. That meant, for instance, that doctors without an infectious disease background were permitted to treat COVID-19 patients in the ICU. Same for nurses who were not trained in critical care. So we employed them as functional nurses, meaning they worked alongside the critical care nurses and performed noncritical nursing care while the critical care nurses performed the more critical decision-making and care.

To adapt to our staffing shortages, we changed to a model called team nursing. It was no longer a one-to-one primary care nursing setup but a more team-based approach. At one point, we constructed a mini pod where there might be six patients, two critical care nurses, and four functional nurses. The critical care nurses handled the major decisions, medications, assessments, and oversight of the functional nurses. Our nurses who were displaced by the focus away from elective surgery and ambulatory care played an important role in caring for the critically ill patients at the height of the crisis.

THE PPE

One of the hardest things to get used to was not seeing the faces of people I had worked with for years. I had always prided myself on learning people's names, looking them in the eye, and getting to know them as much as I could. It wasn't strategic; I truly enjoy people, and I learn something new from everyone I meet. Now, we were all covered from head to toe in PPE, rushing around the unit like an army of alien marshmallows.

Sure, my colleagues were beside me, working every day, but I couldn't actually see them. With the personal protective equipment, only their eyes were visible through their goggles and face shields. It never stopped feeling weird to walk among these swishing clouds of yellow and blue, knowing that my colleagues were in there somewhere. We all felt a little crazy at times. Sometimes, you could tell someone was having a bad day only by seeing the tears spilling out of their eyes through their face shields. And there were plenty of bad days.

We hard to learn to recognize people's eyes. Someone came up with a brilliant idea to print out our ID badges with our pictures magnified to make us more easily recognizable, and that worked. We tried to lighten things up. We made our gowns fancy by wearing colorful hats. Some hats were donated to us, handmade and colorful, and it was so much fun just being distracted by the wild designs. I had a large collection of these hats that I would coordinate with my scrubs; I still have them. I didn't see my hair for months. It was all well and good, as I could not have gotten it professionally done, and I am not very good at doing my own hair.

THE PATIENTS

Monday, March 16, 2020, began a time in my life that I hope I never have to relive. I am saying this with the utmost respect for those who lost loved ones during the pandemic. Personally, I had never experienced death and suffering on such a large scale, and to this day, I find it very difficult to even think about those days. Our patients were the sickest of the sick. None could speak. They were all in isolation rooms and on ventilators. The chaos in my unit and others across the hospital was not a management or staffing problem. All around me, human beings were fighting for their lives, and many of them were losing. And there was very little anyone could do about it.

The patients came to us gasping for air; many were already on ventilators by the time they came to the ICU. For many patients in that first wave, the ventilators did not make much of a difference. The pictures shown on TV of patients gasping for air were difficult to watch, but in real life, it was a horrible experience. To see men and women in that condition within touching distance is not something I'd wish on anyone who hasn't been trained to deal with it. We soon began to run short on regular ventilators and had to retrieve older ventilators from storage that sat on tables next to the patients. Thankfully, we never ran out of PPE or other important supplies as the crisis stretched on over the next several weeks.

Patients coming into the emergency room with respiratory issues were typically given a chest X-ray. One of our doctors described the worst patients' condition as akin to having glue in the lungs. No air was passing through; there was no air exchange for the natural transfer of oxygen through the body because their mucus was so thick. Even on the ventilators, there was no comfortable breathing because the airways were blocked. Bronchoscopy images would show this sticky, gooey, glue-like stuff in the lungs. The patients did not look good, and we were losing them by the hour.

THE HOSPITAL

Loading dock workers are not the typical group one thinks about in conversations and articles about COVID-19. But I did and sometimes still do think about them. At the height of the first wave, the hospital had set up makeshift morgues on the loading dock where supplies normally come into the hospital. These workers, who were not trained medical workers, had to witness hundreds of dead patients being placed into these refrigerated trucks. They had to do their work in an environment that they probably never imagined. It must have been so distressing for them.

A tent was set up on the grounds outside the emergency department, and patients would be treated out there when the emergency department was at capacity. It was an unbelievable scene. Ambulances would be lined up, lights flashing, not able to even get close to the door of the emergency department. At times, patients were treated while in the ambulance.

COUNTING THE LOSSES

We were instructed to take our temperature daily and to monitor ourselves for COVID-19 symptoms. I always felt fine, but the fear was always present. The steadily climbing number of patients of color did not escape my notice. And many of these patients were coming to us very sick, already on ventilators, with comorbidities like diabetes, hypertension, and heart disease. In addition to the seven men I described earlier, I remember one pregnant Black woman. She, too, was intubated and unable to speak or breathe. She passed away, and so did her baby. There were also three middle-aged men of South Asian descent who fought so hard for their lives for days but ultimately lost their battles.

Patients would come into the intensive care unit, and some died right away, while others died after two to three days. By the time they reached the critical care unit in March and April 2020, it was too late for the majority of them.

The public service message at that point was for everyone to stay home and flatten the curve. Terrified families were dropping their loved ones off at the emergency department, saying goodbye, and driving off quickly. We had shut down visitation by then, so the patients were dying isolated, with their families likely terrified at home.

The doctors and nurses began to set up FaceTime calls so that families could at least see the patients on screen. The nurses were the only connection some patients had to their families and loved ones. It didn't make the staff's jobs any easier to have to set up these calls or to witness the pain these families were going through. But it was a welcome means to allow them to communicate with their loved ones.

CHAPTER 20

The Surge and Surge B

Media reports estimated that twenty thousand New Yorkers died of COVID-19 during the peak of April 2020. Whatever the actual numbers were, I can say that I witnessed too many deaths, and I continue to struggle with those images of dying and dead patients to this day.

During the same period, however, we also discharged patients, even some from the ICU. There was no greater joy than seeing a patient emerging from intubation—some after weeks on a ventilator—and breathing on their own, then going home with their families. While each death was difficult, each discharge was celebrated by the staff with gongs, cheers, and streamers. We had to do it; every win was so sweet because there were so, so many losses.

RUNNING OUT OF ROOM

As late April 2020 got underway, the need for more beds posed a constant challenge. I was overwhelmed by an all-consuming sense of emergency.

Everything was just work, sleep, work, sleep. By the time the peak hit, I had even begun to forget my fear of being infected. My team was so busy trying to situate and move critically ill patients. Area hospitals were quickly becoming overwhelmed by patient volume, and it fell to Northwell's integrated hospital system to help them as well as ourselves.

Northwell's leadership implemented a system called "load balancing," in which patients from Northwell's twenty-one hospitals were distributed to any hospital within the system where beds were available to prevent any one hospital from becoming overwhelmed. And the patients kept coming. Typically, the total number of beds in our hospital is a little over 570; that is our occupancy limit. However, during the height of the COVID-19 crisis, we were housing more than nine hundred patients.

When the volume of patients at LIJMC would not let up, we expanded to our capacity in just about every possible area. We had moved from the traditional ICU into our ambulatory care same-day surgery units that had monitors and could safely care for patients. We surged into our post-anesthesia care units and just about everywhere that could accommodate a patient with a monitor.

LIJMC's building is attached to the Cohen Children's Medical Center, and the decision was made to surge into their facility since COVID-19 was not significantly affecting children at that time. It made perfect sense. Cohen Children's Hospital's volume was low, and we were able to capture some of their space both for an ICU unit and to house noncritical patients.

Moving patients is a painstaking, exhausting process. It is physically and mentally taxing to transport seriously ill patients attached to heavy equipment from one facility to another: the pushing and moving of the beds, the care to make sure that all the wires and IVs remain connected and that the patients were not disturbed or harmed, and the careful planning and logistics. It was a soul-wearying project, but we moved ahead.

Unfortunately, we found ourselves having to play musical beds between critical care and medical patients, as the care needs of the patients constantly shifted. One day, we moved several patients into this newly built intensive care unit. But just one week later, we were told we had to move those patients again; the hospital needed the space for lower acuity medicine patients. The groans on my team shook me, and I sympathized with them. Again, we kept our heads down and did the work. It was a constant pushing of beds, lifesaving equipment, including ventilators, and, of course, people. Our strength and patience were being tested to their limits every day.

SURGE B

If you visit the children's hospital on the LIJMC campus, you will see a beautiful lobby with child-friendly decor. Along the walls are orange-, blue-, and green-colored artwork that evokes starfish and aquatic scenes. There is a fish tank in the lobby.

Before COVID-19, there was a nondescript space to the side of that lobby that had been earmarked for pediatric operating and recovery rooms. It was a gray, blank slate, almost industrial-looking, before the construction, logistics, management, and engineers all got to work on what would quickly become a fifty-five-bed intensive care unit that we called Surge B. All of that work came together in just two weeks.

Ask any of the nurses who worked there, and you'll find that they either loved or loathed Surge B. I recently ran into a colleague whom I hadn't seen since 2020, during the height of the pandemic. "Hey!" He called out to me. "Remember me from Surge B?" He was one of the nurses who loved it, and I deeply appreciate his hard work and commitment to this day. To love Surge B, you had to be the kind of person who's a grinder, a tough worker who can tolerate a lot of uncertainty.

Surge B wasn't fancy. Think warehouse, a wide-open space with beds and monitors. And bodies, just bodies, everywhere, lying in beds or walking about covered in PPE. Patient space was a priority, so there was not much room to set up desks, but we wanted the staff situated right next to the patient. For every two beds, we placed computers on wheeled desks plus a chair, and that was the setup. A lot of the traveling nurses ended up working in Surge B, along with physicians taking up extra shifts and the occasional per diem worker.

The entire hospital, from management to the lowest ranks, was committed to making sure we could care for the high volume of critically ill patients. It was a matter of being able to quickly pivot from one plan to a better plan and come up with creative and bold solutions like building out a new unit, retrofitting an unused space, or redirecting patients to another location. We were in a wartime mode.

Surge B, like the other critical care units, was chaotic all day, every day. Busy staff moving around and patients on ventilators and continuous venovenous hemofiltration (CVVH) machines to treat acute kidney failure and stave off permanent kidney damage. Overhead was the constant clatter of emergency alerts being called over the PA system and the phones ringing off the hook. Everybody had questions; people wanted to talk to doctors. Doctors couldn't stop to talk because they were running from bed to bed trying to save lives, or they were in the middle of complicated procedures. It was crazy; that is how I would describe Surge B.

Some nights, it didn't even make sense to go home. Some of the staff rented Airbnbs and hotel rooms or stayed with friends. Nurses came in early, stayed late, and even came in on their days off. I can't say enough how courageous we all were for continuing to show up tired, afraid, and not knowing what was coming next.

THE EMOTIONAL TOLL IN HINDSIGHT

In my memory, Surge B remains a sea of bodies, bodies, and bodies of people, positioned supine or prone, silent and helpless. Beside them were machines and equipment blinking, hissing, and beeping. There were dozens of staff moving around, gowns swishing around, causing a constant echo of soft noise in the crowded, cavernous unit. Neither I nor any of my colleagues had seen or experienced anything like that in our lives. At the time, I didn't stop long enough to think about it, but sometimes, Surge B resurfaces in my memory like a doorway to death.

I still have a mental picture of walking into Surge B and knowing exactly who was in what bed, when they were admitted, and from where. I will probably never shake the images of black men, rows of sick black men isolated in beds, anonymous and silent under breathing tubes and hospital gowns. They all died.

I still have images of a family—a mother, father, son, and daughter—who came into Surge B together and who probably died together.

I still have these images of going into the unit and seeing bodies, dead bodies.

I still have images of pregnant women who died.

I still have images of people who we thought would die but who survived.

I still have images of the first time we closed Surge B.

We created a group, Team Lavender, to give the staff and whoever else wanted to come some closure. We invited chaplains, our holistic nurse, and others to join us for this moment of silence in Surge B. We wanted to honor the people who had died there and their families and to give the staff an opportunity to reflect and grieve.

Unfortunately, we had to reopen Surge B when the omicron variant struck. It was déjà vu—another sea of bodies, another sea of sadness and loss.

We finally closed Surge B in September 2021. We had another ceremony, and my team and I walked through the unit. We invited some survivors to come back, and a few did. One survivor returned with his entire family and spoke at the ceremony.

As my team of leaders, managers, and assistant nurse managers walked through the unit for the last time, the tears flowed. We needed that time to be there again in that empty space where we saw and experienced so much loss. Walking together as a team helped ease the pain for me because I knew I was not alone in what I was feeling.

CHAPTER 21

Good Times, Bad Times

The first wave went on from early March until around late May 2020. Since early May, the messages from hospital leadership, and even the media, were encouraging to a degree. We'd heard about COVID-19 tests that would soon be available to the public. Word was also getting around that the CDC was working with pharmaceutical companies on a vaccine that could be available before the year was over. Moreover, some of the medical therapies were working, and more drugs were being promised. Non-pharmaceutical interventions were also proving effective as the caseloads dropped with mandatory stay-at-home orders and increased use of masks across the country. After the chaos and misery of the April surge, hope was slowly blooming. Around the early summer, we began to see a break, as the number of patients dying began to slow down and more patients began to survive COVID-19, going home to their families.

Here are some data from a CDC report[26] that gives an idea of what we were up against during those first few months of the pandemic:

- From February 29, 2020, to June 1, 2020, a total of 203,792 COVID-19 cases were diagnosed and reported among residents of New York City.
- 54,211 (26.6 percent) known to have been hospitalized.
- 18,679 (9.2 percent) died.
- Among hospitalized patients, 32.1 percent were known to have died.

The CDC report noted that during those months, case counts increased rapidly from a weekly mean of 274 diagnosed cases per day during the week of March 8 to a peak weekly mean of 5,132 cases per day by the week of March 29. The median duration of hospitalization was six days.

WE HAD A JOB TO DO

During the first wave, we were exposed to death on a scale that none of us had ever experienced. To say that we were traumatized would be a cliché and understatement. When I heard of longtime nurses and doctors walking away from the profession during those months, I understood. We entered the profession to help people, not to watch them die in the dozens every week. I can't say that my early training in the oncology unit prepared me for this because, in terms of the number of patients, their ages, and the seeming randomness of the virus in who lived or died, there just was no comparison. Not even close.

Throughout all the deaths and suffering, my staff and I were determined to keep working, to keep fighting for our patients. We worked sixteen-hour days multiple times, seven days a week. Even when home, my phone would constantly be ringing. Staffing plans were complicated;

---

[26] Corinne N. Thompson et al., "CDC Morbidity and Mortality Report: COVID-19 Outbreak — New York City, February 29–June 1, 2020," *Morbidity and Mortality Weekly Report*, 69, no. 46 (2020): 1725–29, http://dx.doi.org/10.15585/mmwr.mm6946a2.

it was like moving pieces around on a chessboard. At some point, I began to consciously apply my academic training and experience in leadership and nursing to what was happening at the hospital. Thankfully, I was not doing this alone. I had a strong team of nurse managers and assistant nurse managers providing constant support. At one point, we simply rearranged the leadership assignments so that we had one person focused only on the staff, making (and negotiating) schedules, making assignments, and that sort of thing. Anne, who was pregnant at the time, did a phenomenal job with playing staffing chess, although most days, I thought she wanted to kill me. I did my best to keep her stress level as low as possible.

One day, Anne was sitting with me in my office. I had recently put her in charge of onboarding the traveling nurses. She looked around my office, observing the dozens of pairs of shoes lined up along the walls. "Wow," she said. "You just have all these shoes here picking up dust?" I took that as a challenge. There I was, wearing high heels and scrubs that morning—albeit for just a couple of minutes. We had a great laugh at that, but it felt empowering, as if COVID-19 hadn't completely robbed all the joy out of our lives.

At one point, I decided to start fighting back by doing little things I enjoyed, even though they didn't make a whole lot of sense. One day, I was going home, and Anne noticed me putting on lipstick. "You know you're going to have to put on that mask, right?" Dang! I didn't need to hear that kind of truth in that moment. But wearing lipstick even for a few moments made me feel like pre-COVID-19 me, and it felt good!

Across the board, the staff was putting on a courageous fight every day. But they were human. Some days, it was too much, and people were too sick and wisely stayed home. Leadership always needed to have a Plan A, Plan B, and Plan C to staff those shifts. Some days, my nurse managers and I were gratefully surprised when more people showed up than we expected. Traveling workers were a godsend! Our leadership team did their job effectively and learned to adapt quickly. Every day, I thought, "I work with an amazing group of people!"

Occasionally, if we saw a team member fading, we told them to go home or that it was okay to take the next day to recharge. We needed everyone to stay healthy. This level of team cohesion brought me back to my early years as a nurse in the oncology unit at Lenox Hill. When you work in difficult situations with very sick patients, you need a tight team that is not only empathetic to the patients but to their colleagues as well.

I mentioned earlier my colleague Paul, who was one of the few people who adapted well to working in Surge B. I can't give this guy enough credit for his work ethic and wonderful personality. He left Northwell and moved South in 2021, and it's the hospital's loss. When I ran into him in 2023, he was still upbeat about the work we did in Surge B. "We had some good times in there, Sandra." When no one wanted to take the reins and lead that area, Paul stepped up and did a phenomenal job. He is among dozens of nurses and colleagues I could name here who gave completely of themselves during the height of the crisis to care for our patients and keep their colleagues motivated.

When staff members did get sick, they felt guilty. The Northwell policy required staffers to quarantine for fourteen days until they were symptom-free. Several of our nursing staff who did become infected and were home sick would call in to work to check on their colleagues. Some of our team members said they couldn't wait to come back to work.

SHARING THE BURDEN

During the first wave, there was this adrenaline, and we all went into overdrive. We wanted to be there in the thick of the action, fighting the virus and taking care of our patients. No one wanted to get sick and have their colleagues deal with the chaos on the floor. So there was this guilt. We desperately wanted to remain in the fight against this horrible virus. Yes, at times, we felt afraid for ourselves and our families, but the most powerful feeling on our team was our desire to fight and win the battle against COVID-19.

On any given day, the staff had so many questions. I remember going into one of the units one Sunday, and a swarm of staff descended on me.

They were so scared, and they had so many questions and requests. Some lived at home with older parents and were terrified of bringing home the virus. The deaths we were seeing on a daily basis in the hospital haunted us. Would our families be next? Would we be next?

Sometimes, the fear clothed itself in practical issues. Why couldn't the nurses have showers available at work so they could shower before going home? Why couldn't there be more scrubs to change in and out of after exposure to patients? Many times, I didn't have answers for them. But I listened to each request and tried to be as transparent as possible. Most times, my answer was, "I don't know, but I'll look it up," or "I can make that request for you."

I remember one nurse who was young and not very experienced, probably about two years into his career at the hospital. During one shift, I could see he was struggling, so I approached him. My instinct was confirmed. He had never experienced a patient dying and had never done postmortem care. "Come," I told him. "Let's do this together." We went through the process together, and I could sense his appreciation. We sent the patient to the morgue, and there was no relief or happiness in that, but we did it together and moved on to the next challenge.

My goal was to be visible, accessible, and involved. While I didn't have a one-to-one patient assignment, I felt a sense of ownership over every facet of the work in the ICUs. I fetched equipment, PPE, lunch, supplies, and whatever the staff needed. Months after the first wave, I received a beautiful handwritten thank-you note with a Starbucks gift card from Marie, a nurse who remembered how I walked all over the hospital to get her a piece of equipment and hand-delivered it to her. Her kindness brought me to tears. I helped cover snack breaks (most days, a full break was unheard of), and I cleaned up and organized supplies. These might seem like menial tasks but, trust me, I was honored to be serving my staff in these little ways.

We conducted a staff satisfaction survey shortly after the crisis abated in 2021. I expected terrible results; I could tell it was going to be a disaster. Surprisingly, it wasn't. Management received high satisfaction scores from the staff. Several people in management did not think it was a good idea to do a staff survey after a time of so much chaos and uncertainty. But I am glad we did it. My thinking was whatever the results were, we would learn from it and commit to doing better.

CHAPTER 22

Summer of 2020

I was finishing up my doctorate during COVID-19, and frankly, the research work was a welcome distraction on my infrequent off days, late at night, and the wee hours of the morning before going into the hospital. Scheduling my research assignments on my off days made me feel hopeful, like there was a future worth working toward that didn't involve COVID-19.

As overwhelming as work had become, I didn't always look forward to coming home. The lockdowns had turned New York into a dystopian wasteland, deserted and quiet, way too quiet. The things I loved about the city—the energy, the noise, the people—were nowhere to be found. My drive to work was eerily quick; there were no other cars on the street and no one honking at me to step on it when the light turned green. The drive home was lonely, especially after a long day of being surrounded by colleagues and patients.

The outside world just felt strange. It was spring, and flowers were blooming, but I couldn't enjoy it. I wasn't focused on what I was going to plant for the summer or planning to visit the garden store for soil and gardening supplies with my friend Pauline. There was no one walking the streets in the morning when I left for work or returned late at night.

Mom was living by herself in the Bronx, and I was afraid for her because she loved to go out. Would her friends pressure her to go out? Would she remember to always wear a mask, wash her hands, and not let anyone into her house? My mom, in her old age, has made many friends and has a rich social life; I worried about what effect the lockdown would have on her mental state. We stayed in touch, though. She would call and check up on me every day. Every couple of days, I would drive by her place to replenish her mask supplies. I would roll the car window down just enough to push the bag through, and that was it. Mom, being Mom, would always slip me a bag of food.

PROTEST SUMMER

The campus at LIJMC is beautiful. New Hyde Park, where the hospital is located, is a pleasant suburb with mature trees that add some life to the office parks that line the edge of the neighborhoods. To get away from the chaos of work, my team and I took walks around the hospital campus when we could. We laughed, cried, and walked silently sometimes. After a while, we began to make these walks educational and discussed leadership lessons. We called them leadership walk-and-chats. We scheduled them on the calendar because they meant so much to us, to be able to just be with each other, away from the plague. We started at the main entrance and walked around the back of the building, past the emergency department, the loading dock, the older behavioral health hospital building, and into the surrounding neighborhood. It could be a good thirty- to forty-five-minute walk when we turned back into the Cohen Children's Hospital lobby. We grew more and more comfortable sharing our vulnerability, and these times brought us closer together as a team.

On these walks, we did our best not to talk about what was happening on the floor. Instead, we would just talk and try to joke around and get our heads out of the hospital and our faces into the sunlight. Getting out into the world, so to speak, did wonders for our perspective and replenished our emotional energy.

Around early June, our walks became a little tense as the protests over the George Floyd murder grew more widespread. For months, the media images from the Internet and television had been focused on the pandemic, the death tolls, the testing controversies, and the political controversies. But after the George Floyd video was made public in late May, the world seemed to explode. No one could ignore the scenes of hurt, rage, and protest across the country that were being broadcast on the news daily. Hospitals, major corporations, academic institutions, and other major institutions were making broad statements on their commitment to racial justice and against police brutality.

Our team is diverse, with members from around the world, and as a manager, I had to be careful about my words. Some of our team members were married to police officers, and I could sense their tension at times. I wanted to make sure my team felt free to speak—or not feel pressured to speak—their minds. We needed to be inclusive but in a holistic way. I wanted my team to be sensitive and not label all police officers as bad people, like the ones involved in George Floyd's killing. I didn't want my colleagues whose spouses were police officers to feel guilty or that I was angry with them personally for any reason. I wanted us to be able to talk about it and for them to know that I know the difference between a bad police officer and a good police officer. We had a conversation, and I thought it was respectful, and I'm happy I did it. We weren't walking around with uncertainty or walking on eggshells around each other. I addressed the concept of being inclusive as an opportunity to expand even further to make sure that all our nurses feel like they, too, were part of that inclusiveness.

As a leader, I had my own thoughts and concerns. I was shocked by the killing of George Floyd and felt so angry, disempowered, and at a complete loss at times. I spoke to my son and my brother often during those days to make sure they were okay. They were both resigned yet hurt, so hurt by the image of that police officer's knee on Floyd's neck for nearly nine minutes—it could have been either of them. From talking with my friends and family, we all felt despondent for weeks, some longer. Combined with the losses from COVID-19, there was just a collective burden weighing us down for the remainder of 2020.

FEELING MY FEELINGS WHILE LEADING

The hospital held events to give the staff an opportunity to grieve, talk about their experiences, and express solidarity with social justice movements. Our CEO was encouraging and supportive. I remember one ceremony we held on the grounds of LIJMC where dozens of people kneeled together. These events brought the staff together in so many good ways, and I appreciated being a part of them.

But there was a deep sense of sadness that I think people of color were feeling. It was part disappointment that this type of brazen brutality could still happen in the twenty-first century. It was also a sense of powerlessness over the fact that, since at least Trayvon Martin, no amount of protest seemed to be preventing these sorts of deadly incidents from recurring. As always, my family was my rock during this time as we shared our grief, shock, and anger in endless conversations.

Honestly, I did not want to share those feelings with my team. I am sharing them publicly now, of course. But at the time, I didn't think it was appropriate to discuss my personal feelings at work in that way. I wanted to remain levelheaded and strong so that my staff could come to me if they needed to vent or just needed someone to listen.

For better or worse, my personal ethos has always been to leave my personal stress at home as much as possible. If my problems were very serious, I did let my boss know, and I would take the time off that I needed. That is more of a personality issue than a leadership tactic or strategy.

I still believe that as leaders and managers, we have to be careful about how we talk about controversial or sensitive issues. Not all members of our staff are in the same political, social, or even age demographic. We won't always be right, but we can be caring. We are human, and we are never going to please everyone; that is just reality. But in the workplace, we owe it to our people to be measured and thoughtful in our words and reactions whenever possible. Thankfully, there were no major disagreements on my team, although not everyone was in agreement with some of the statements being made at the hospital level.

Leadership is tough, but leading through a pandemic layered with social and political conflict is tougher. On some of the tougher days, I would come home some nights and dream of all the other things I could be doing with my life: living on a farm, growing produce, raising chickens, and wearing overalls. I could do a lot more traveling. I wondered if I would ever get a chance to do those things.

So, while people of all backgrounds broke out of lockdown and rallied into the streets of New York and across the country to protest, I went to work. The death rates were falling, and we were seeing more discharges, but the feeling of heaviness stuck with me. The social unrest and the feeling of hopelessness about race relations did not help.

Some days, I woke up and lay in bed; I didn't want to get dressed; I had nothing left to give to the world. As you know by now, I am quite a clotheshorse, but during that summer, I wore the same black outfit most days.

COVID-19 was bringing me down with it. The few moments in a day that I took to reflect brought more fear and anxiety. I would turn on the news, and the death counts would be on the screen, with the estimated deaths for the next week. Those estimates would be shattering after a day of work in the ICU. All I would recall were the patients who looked like me, black people, men and women, suffering and dying, alone and silent.

The news reporter would report that the CDC was expecting two hundred thousand more deaths, and I thought, "Oh, God! Is that me? Is that my family member? Who are these other 200,000 people who will die in the next few weeks?" I did end up losing two family members to COVID-19: my aunt, who was in her seventies, and another elderly uncle.

I was never a big believer in psychotherapy. I grew up in a family that believed in just working hard and not thinking too hard about problems.

Our hospital made available to the staff counseling and other services to help them cope with the trauma and stress. There were reflecting rooms, on-site chapels, and the like. I had to work through my skepticism and admit that I needed the help I was encouraging my staff to accept. Experts from Northwell's Center for Traumatic Stress Resilience and Recovery educated us on tools and strategies to build resilience and deal with stress and trauma. The program was effective, and I am glad I participated in it. I highly recommend that anyone still struggling with the difficulties of the pandemic or the effects of racial or other kinds of trauma seek help from a medical professional. It is a worthwhile and absolute blessing to have this type of care.

CHAPTER 23

Here Comes the Sun

There were days when all we could do as a staff was laugh with and at one another. One day, I took a long look at myself in the mirror. There I was, wearing scrubs and clogs again, masked up to my eyes. The last time I had worn heels to work was months ago, on March 13, 2020. Some days, I got so sick of the drab image that I would have a desire to wear something cute to work. But the reality was not cute, and I had to face it in scrubs.

One day, after the first big wave and during a bit of a lull, I tried to muster up the strength to put an outfit together. As soon as I walked into the surgical intensive care unit, one of the nurses and the nurse manager looked me up and down. "Where are you going, Sandra? Why are you all dressed up?" I had become one of them by wearing scrubs. They loved to see me in scrubs. I reassured them that I was not leaving them. I just needed to get out of the rut I was in.

BEYOND THE WAVE

The support from the community had been so inspiring to us during the spring. It was not like the daily pots banging and yelling like you saw on the news in New York City, but we were celebrated in our Queens community. The fire department would come out at the end of the shifts every day to cheer us on, and we received tons of donations of food every single day. I've never seen so many pizza pies in my life! We also had top-line chefs from the fanciest restaurants sending us meals; one restaurant even created an ice cream bar for us. The love we felt from the Greater New York area and beyond was so beautiful and overwhelming.

We began to adapt to our new normal. Our nurses, as well as the community, began to show their creative side. People would make us colorful hats and hats with crazy prints or designs. It began to be a way for us to identify one another. We were all covered in personal protective equipment from head to toe, but your colleagues could know you from the hat you were wearing. Some of the staff also began to make giant pictures and badges out of their ID photos and wore those on their PPE so we could tell who was who. By the time May rolled around and the cases began to subside a bit, we had become more battle-tested and confident.

I'll also never forget the tailgate parties that some of the staff members threw. These parties would not be at the hospital, of course. Word would spread (the staff is very much on social media, by the way) that folks would be meeting in a Walmart parking lot after the shift. Beers would be cracked open, and there would be lots of commiserating, laughter, silliness, and lots of blowing off steam. The tailgating became such a thing that some of our nurses would always keep a cooler in the trunk or the hatchback for these parties that helped us decompress after a tough week. They were always safe, outdoors and away from the general public.

The biggest celebrations we had, however, were over our patients who beat the virus and were discharged. There would be a clap out for each patient all the way to their waiting transportation. When a patient was taken off a ventilator, everyone would hear "Here Comes the Sun" over the PA system. It was a beautiful sound in those late spring days when we began to see more and more patients improve. By then, there were more therapies, such as Remdesivir, dexamethasone, and antibody treatments. We were starting to see good results, and that song heralded hope across the hospital.

On a personal level, I tried to recognize my staff for their courage and commitment whenever I could. I always made sure to thank them for agreeing to work an extra shift. I made sure they saw me rolling up my sleeves right alongside them and not aloof and away from the patients. That meant making sure they had what they needed to do their jobs and being that throughline to management—a trustworthy advocate for them—when questions and issues arose.

Our hospital was among many giving nurses $1,000 and $2,500 bonuses plus additional time off. While I couldn't personally give them bonuses, I made sure their needs were addressed. For example, many staff were concerned about bringing the virus home to their families after a day on the wards. We instituted a scrub exchange program where there was a place where uniforms could be changed after shifts or the nurses could shower and change. We also had central areas set aside for eating or taking a break. One place that was sacred and would not be considered for ICU beds was the cafeteria. Hospital leadership rightly felt that the staff needed a place that felt like their own where they could get away from the chaos of the patient wards.

THE OMICRON WAVE

When omicron struck in the late summer and fall of 2021, we were only slightly better prepared. While we had learned some things from the first wave, there was still a struggle to understand the virus because things were changing so quickly; for one thing, omicron was a different strain than the delta strain of the first wave. As it became clearer that omicron was even more contagious than delta, the old fears, panic, and chaos began to rear their heads again.

We had the space for patients. Our challenge was getting the staff to deal with the patient surge. Our team was back to begging nurses and staff to work overtime. We tried to do a better job this time of keeping the staff healthy and keeping ourselves from experiencing burnout. But by then, many nurses were beginning to quit the profession or just work less. They were exhausted, disillusioned, and still coping with the grief and trauma from the first wave.

It wasn't just the nurses who were leaving the profession. After the first wave, physicians, administrators, orderlies, PCAs, and staff across all disciplines were burnt out. Many walked away from the profession, saying that this was not what they signed up for. Some nurses went to work in doctors' offices, some went to ambulatory care sites or took early retirement, and some left the profession altogether. Our leadership was back to competing with other hospitals for the same small pool of traveling nurses.

There were new treatments in development, and some were getting more media attention than was warranted. Monoclonal antibodies, for instance, were making the news headlines, but only a small number of people were able to get access to that treatment. The treatment made a significant difference in terms of reducing the length of hospitalizations, and patients reported that they felt stronger and better able to withstand the effects of the virus. Some of my colleagues received monoclonal antibodies and saw improved outcomes. But I will note the difficulty of even getting an appointment for most people. There were few health-care locations offering monoclonal antibody treatments, so it was far from widely available. The barriers were high; patients had to meet certain criteria before they could qualify. So, while it was encouraging that this treatment was offering up some good results, the majority of patients would not have access.

Omicron dominated my life for several months into 2022. But then other demands started to pull on me. The requirements of my vaccine advocacy work began to increase, raising a whole new set of stresses. I was battered and beaten and bruised from the many waves of the virus and my day job of leading the critical care division. And I was now being thrust into the spotlight and advocating for vaccine awareness and equity.

CHAPTER 24

On Nursing and Burnout

We hug. Sometimes, we cry. We share pictures of grandkids, a wedding, or a new dog or cat. We follow each other on social media and tease one another about the latest vacation pictures. We share when we move houses or buy a new car or adopt a new pet. It is so wonderful to catch up with these lovely men and women who make up the nursing staff at Northwell and who together worked through and experienced the worst of the pandemic. We are from a variety of backgrounds: Black immigrant, Asian, Caucasian, African American. This battle-tested group of professionals continues to be committed to their work caring for patients every day. We all are recovering still, trying to move on with our lives, and grateful to still be doing what we love.

However, not all nurses across the US are doing well. It may take years before some feel well enough to reenter the nursing profession—if they ever do. I know a few experienced nurses who took early retirement and some newly minted nurses who decided that the profession wasn't for them. I understand and empathize with their exhaustion and disillusionment. I feel for the nurses who developed post-traumatic stress syndrome and are still trying to recover their mental health.

A *New York Times* article[27] recently listed some reasons for nurses' predicament: the increase in patient deaths during the pandemic, a shortage of workers leading to understaffing, and increased violence toward health-care workers over masking mandates. These are nation-wide problems that will impact the nursing profession for years to come. When I speak with nurses who continue to face these challenges up close and personal, I worry for the future of the profession.

STRESS AND BURNOUT

Even before the pandemic, nurses reported burnout and fatigue due to staffing shortages. COVID-19 only worsened the existing problems. Nearly 100,000 US registered nurses left the profession during the pandemic, and 610,000 registered nurses said they had an "intent to leave" the workforce by 2027, according to a study from the National Council of State Boards of Nursing,[28] which cites stress and burnout as the main causes. In the same study, the council found a quarter to half of nurses reported feeling emotionally drained (50.8 percent), used up (56.4 percent), fatigued (49.7 percent), burned out (45.1 percent), or at the end of the rope (29.4 percent) "a few times a week" or "every day." The council's report states that with a quarter of the population contemplating leaving the profession, the impact of the pandemic may be felt way into the future.

Critical care nurses were particularly more susceptible to burnout than nurses in other disciplines. Before the pandemic, we would probably experience one or two ICU deaths a week. Even as an experienced nurse who worked for years in an oncology unit, it was rare to see more

---

[27] Bradford Pearson, "Nurses Are Burned Out. Can Hospitals Change in Time to Keep Them?" *New York Times*, February 20, 2023, https://www.nytimes.com/2023/02/20/well/nurses-burnout-pandemic-stress.html.

[28] "Nursing at the Crossroads: A Call to Action," National Council of State Boards of Nursing, Inc, 2023, https://www.ncsbn.org/video/nursing-at-the-crossroads.

than a few patient deaths in a single week. COVID-19, however, turned all those expectations on their heads. At the height of the crisis, we could see a dozen deaths per day. The sheer volume of patients and their dire condition—intubated, lying on their stomachs, swollen, and unable to speak—was a source of trauma for many nurses. Then, there was our own fear of getting infected and bringing the virus home to our families. Add to that all of the social unrest of the summer of 2020. Among the millions of protesters across the nation were doctors and nurses who also publicly stood against racial injustice even while facing enormous amounts of work stress.

IN HER OWN WORDS

Critical care nurses were not the only ones facing extraordinary stress and burnout during COVID-19. Nurses who provided care to the elderly and other ill patients also had to deal with the unique challenges brought on by the virus.

W.P. is a veteran nurse who works with elderly patients in a mid-size town in a Southern state. While W.P. credits her institution for being quick to adopt safety measures when the pandemic struck, she observed that the patients and the surrounding community were not as quick to acknowledge the seriousness of COVID-19. This lack of buy-in from the community led to serious challenges in her workplace. She related some of her experiences below.

- I work with elderly patients, and they can be very belligerent at times. I've been grabbed, pushed, and struck by angry patients, even before COVID-19. But during COVID-19, things got worse. One night, I was working late, and one of my patients was this angry man who kept swearing up and down that he didn't have COVID-19. He was already very sick, and then he became infected with COVID-19 on top of that. His family couldn't do anything with him. This guy pulled out his PICC line (a PICC line delivers fluid to the body intravenously) and got very physical with me. There was blood everywhere! Luckily, a couple of orderlies came to help, and I could walk away and collect myself.

- I feel that COVID-19 not only made people physically ill, but it also brought out so much mental illness. People were really acting out more than you would normally see. Some people were basically falling apart, physically and emotionally. And during COVID-19, that's what happened. I think the patients who were in denial were the hardest to deal with. It was hard to keep them calm at times. They were just not very accepting. They didn't want to be isolated or be told that there was no more family visitation and that kind of thing.

- For the elderly patients who were sick and isolated, it was very difficult. As people were dying from the virus, they couldn't have family come in to do the social rituals of spending time with them toward the end. That is very important to people in those smaller towns in my area.

- It hurts us, too, as nurses. We formed bonds with some of the patients and knew their families. So it was hard. We didn't have the closure of a funeral or the pleasure of sharing words of tribute to this person who had lived a long life. It just wasn't the same doing it through the website. Down here, people are used to big family funerals, so people didn't have that kind of closure.

FACING DISCRIMINATION AT WORK

In addition to the normal stresses of day-to-day nursing, nurses of color also can face bias from patients, colleagues, and supervisors. A little over 6 percent of nurses identify as Black/African American, according to the 2022 National Nursing Workforce Survey released by the NCSBN and the National Forum of State Nursing Workforce Centers.[29] I found that

---

[29] Kechi Iheduru-Anderson, "Barriers to Career Advancement in the Nursing Profession: Perceptions of Black Nurses in the United States," *Nursing Forum*, 55, no. 4 (July 8, 2020), https://doi.org/10.1111/nuf.12483.

number to be surprisingly low. Living in New York City gives me the advantage of being around a diverse population. But that is not the case for the majority of nurses around the country.

A 2020 study on race in the nursing profession found that "Black nurses face significant challenges in entering leadership or faculty positions." These challenges included racial discrimination and a lack of access to mentors. As I recounted earlier, it is not easy to become a nurse. The education and focus necessary are not for people who want the easy way out. Plus, nurses are called to care for people in intimate ways: changing their dressings or inserting a catheter, for instance. Not everyone is built for that sort of thing. And then you have the once-in-a-lifetime events like COVID-19, where nurses were exposed to death on an unprecedented scale. All nurses need support. Nurses of color, however, who may face discrimination, need to know that they are valuable to their institutions.

I am grateful for the mentors who helped me along my career path. I am particularly thankful for the men and women of color who inspired me just by showing up and doing the work every day. Representation matters! Seeing doctors and nurses of color encouraged me to keep going during difficult times at work. I remember, as a young nurse fresh out of school, feeling deflated when a patient looked at me in disgust and snapped, "This place is changing." He was referring to the Upper East Side hospital whose staff in the past had been predominantly white. If it were not for other supportive nurses—of all ethnic backgrounds—those types of comments could easily have worn me down over the years and kept me from advancing in my career.

Addressing discrimination and disparities in the nursing profession is a complex battle. It requires people of all backgrounds to come together as allies to call out injustices and demand that organizations address the disparities in measurable ways. We must hold our organizations accountable to ensure that the workforce from the C-suite down is representative of the people they lead and the communities they care for. So, when a patient says, "This place is changing," we can respond, "Yes. For the better!"

As I've said earlier, we need to approach inclusiveness in a more holistic way. For instance, when we hand out challenging assignments or opportunities that expose staff to more influential and senior leaders at Northwell we should look out for the quieter, introverted nurse who performs well but may not be as loud or assertive as our typical go-to staffers. We should take into account a broader portfolio of personal and professional strengths when deciding who will move up into leadership. I am almost certain that there is a well of untapped talent in our hospitals that we have yet to discover.

Other measures institutions can take include implicit bias training; educating staff on diversity, inclusion, and cultural competencies; and engaging in community outreach and education to build trust in the communities they serve.

IN HER OWN WORDS

S.D., a nurse practitioner who specializes in psychology and does talk therapy, can recount several times when meeting a patient in person that they expressed shock at seeing her behind the desk.

- Sometimes, before even getting into why they are there to see me, they want to know where I went to school, about my education, and my professional background. I have gotten used to it over the years. But for some patients, I've had to have their provider find them another nurse practitioner when I find that their attitude will get in the way of the care.
- Then there's the discrimination from colleagues and supervisors. There was always this implication that I had to prove I belonged there. I left one very prestigious job for that reason. It was just too much every day—the constant questions and the feeling that you were always under extra scrutiny. My nursing colleagues who were not minorities never seemed to be asked these questions about where they had gone to school or the kind

of experiences they'd had. Their work would not be scrutinized or double-checked the way mine was. It wasn't worth it.

SUPPORTING ONE ANOTHER

Fortunately, we have a diverse staff at Northwell. That diversity may have a lot to do with where we are located—in the New York metro area. But I do acknowledge the need for more nurses of color, and that is part of my advocacy work now, encouraging young women to consider nursing as a career. There are opportunities for us in the profession to keep those attrition numbers down. As nurse managers and leaders, we could do a better job of supporting and looking out for our colleagues. As older nurses, we can mentor the younger generation of nurses. For those of us near or at retirement, we can consider teaching part-time at a community college or doing some community work where we pass down our knowledge and experiences. Building community is so important, and there are several ways to do so. No nurse should be an island! We can get involved in organizations that support nurses of color, such as the National Black Nurse Practitioner Association and the Black Nurses Association.

MENTORS ARE IMPORTANT

Luckily, I have had some good allies and mentors who have been instrumental in keeping my career moving forward. Many years ago, while I was at Lenox Hill, we had just finished a relatively successful Joint Commission survey, and the senior leadership team at Lenox Hill Hospital was coming around with ice cream sandwiches as a treat. The Joint Commission is the national body that inspects hospitals for compliance and safety.

I introduced myself to the hospital's senior leadership as the nurse manager of the medical ICU, and one woman on the team, Linda, immediately got my attention. "It is such a pleasure to meet you," she said. "My name is Linda, and I would love to mentor you." Linda is a sophisticated white woman who is always well put together. I was blown away. No one had made such an offer before, so I took her up on it. I had sought out leadership coaches before and gave up on that idea when I heard the price tag. Linda became my very own mentor, and we connected over our shared love of gardening and the finer things in life, including high-quality stationery. Linda gave me my first journal, which I still write in today.

Over the years, I added more mentors, formal and informal. I'd also consider my preceptors, who taught me new skills as I moved from one area of nursing to another, as mentors. Among my best and ever-constant mentors is Garfield. He helped me to get started in nursing school and was my biggest and fiercest competitor during graduate school when we had classes together. He has always pushed me to do better and has been here to bounce ideas off and comfort me during tough times.

To whom much is given, much is expected. In addition to seeing the importance of paying it forward, I enjoy teaching and mentoring. After moving along the continuum from novice to expert nurse, I had the opportunity to precept and mentor many nurses, some of whom I still keep in touch with today. I met with my nurse managers leaders one-on-one monthly to discuss their professional development. I also serve as a mentor to several women both inside and outside of Northwell.

FEEDING THE PIPELINE

How can we work toward improving representation? By mentoring the younger generation, supporting the current generation, and promoting nursing as a profession.

I recently interviewed high school students on Northwell Health's podcast, *20-Minute Health Talk*. The students were part of a New York City program called FutureReadyNYC that offers internships to high schoolers. Northwell is a FutureReadyNYC partner, and the youths I interviewed are excited to join the medical profession one day. It was so encouraging to hear them talk intelligently about what they experienced in the hospital, whether it was witnessing a surgery or observing a psychiatric patient ward. That exposure gave those young people something to envision for the future. We need more of these programs across the country and more kids to know that such programs are available to them. That way, we can, from a young age, begin to train and prepare the next generation of nurses and health-care workers.

Northwell is also great at providing training and development for nurses and has innovative ways of addressing staffing needs. Northwell, as an integrated hospital system, is fortunate to have its own nursing agency, which provides flex staff when needed. The flex staff pool not only fills staffing needs but also gives our nurses the opportunity to make extra money by picking up extra shifts at any of our other hospitals.

Health-care systems and organizations can also lower the barriers to entry by hiring more nurses with associate degrees and creating more training and education within their organizations.

CARING FOR OURSELVES AND OTHERS

Over the last three years, "compassion fatigue" has been a common topic on podcasts and in the public conversation on health-care workers, particularly in the aftermath of the pandemic. I believe compassion fatigue is a very real thing for caregivers, even non-nurses. How can we properly care for others when we are too burned out to actually care? It is important that we take charge of our own health and recognize when it is time to reassess and make a change, take a sabbatical, or take a permanent separation from our careers.

I never seriously considered leaving nursing. But I did have my days. The fatigue, despair, and anger at the pandemic made for some terrible days. However, the devastation of COVID-19 only reinforced for me how important nurses were to patient care and how much our communities needed caregivers who looked like them. My job has changed significantly from being a bedside nurse. I am now an advocate and health-care executive with a doctorate, but I do still consider myself a nurse. That had been my dream when I was a little girl, and I am simply not going to walk away from it.

My advice to nurses facing burnout is to put yourself first. Take time off or switch to another area of nursing. It is absolutely an urgent necessity to take care of yourself first.

Part IV

WHAT WE ARE UP AGAINST

CHAPTER 25

A History of Mistrust

To this day, I am still learning about the history of Clarendon, which was the site of several sugar plantations, a major slave rebellion in the seventeenth century, and centuries later, Jamaica's bauxite mining industry. What that land means to me personally is home. Even though I love my garden here in America (and I do spend a lot of time in it), I will always miss the fertile earth, the greenness of where I grew up, and the freshness of everything—clean rain, clear rivers, and bright blue skies nearly every day. The smell of the grass, the taste of sweet, warm cow's milk, and the sound of a river flowing are just some of the things that will forever tie my heart to Clarendon. I can never be away for too long, and I love my house in Jamaica as much as I love my New York home. Despite the development over the last few decades, there are still glimpses of the old pastoral quality that keeps calling me back.

How different that land must have been to the enslaved people who were brought there from Africa a few hundred years before my grandparents settled on their land in Palmers Cross. I doubt these frightened people felt the same love for the land. They maybe saw it as an enemy, a place of suffering. It might have taken hundreds of years for them to identify with it, to love it, as we Jamaicans now fiercely love our beautiful island.

History is complicated and messy. I'm glad my brother inspires me every day to not shy away from it, because knowing the past has helped me understand the present.

THE GUINEA PIG QUESTION

Around the time that the vaccines were being introduced, one could find many public discussions on vaccine hesitancy in the Black community and the history of people of color being exploited in medical experiments by both government and private actors. There were people asking: Why must the first person be a Black woman? Isn't that just adding to the history of Black exploitation, like the Tuskegee Experiment, Henrietta Lacks, and the experiments on Black women by Dr. James Marion Sims?[30]

The truth is, I was not thinking about historical injustices at that time in 2020. I was thinking about life and death, probably a little shell-shocked from working long days and nights, seeing COVID-19 claim hundreds of lives before my eyes over weeks and weeks of misery. Right before my own eyes, families were torn apart from their loved ones, unable to say goodbye in those last moments. I lost an aunt and uncle to

---

[30] "The U.S. Public Health Service (USPHS) Untreated Syphilis Study at Tuskegee was conducted between 1932 and 1972 to observe the natural history of untreated syphilis" among hundreds of Black men. "As part of the study, researchers did not collect informed consent from participants and they did not offer treatment, even after it was widely available. The study ended in 1972 on the recommendation of an Ad Hoc Advisory Panel." — "The USPHS Untreated Syphilis Study at Tuskegee," Centers for Disease Control and Prevention, https://www.cdc.gov/tuskegee/index.html.

Dr. James Marion Sims was a physician who practiced in Alabama during the 1840s. While he has been honored for several advances in women's gynecological treatment, he is also known for conducting inhumane and brutal experiments on enslaved women. — Harriet A. Washington, *Medical Apartheid: The Dark History of Medical Experimentation on Black Americans from Colonial Times to the Present*, Vintage, 2006.

the virus. I saw myself as someone engaged in a battle against a deadly enemy, and I wanted to win.

I was not the only person who got vaccinated on that historical day in December 2020. Several of my colleagues at Northwell would have felt privileged to be among the first batch of employees to receive the Pfizer-BioNTech vaccine. I just happened to be the first in that chair.

Now that the dust has somewhat settled, I can recall fleeting thoughts and doubts I had at the time. And, yes, I remember the shouting media pundits and the toxic political rhetoric. But those headlines and media controversies were never a real concern. I mainly cared about the lives of the people who were coming through the doors of my hospital daily.

Since then, I (like many others) have been on a journey of learning about our past, particularly in the wake of the killing of George Floyd in Minnesota in the summer of 2020. That devastating video only compounded the exhaustion and frustration of what I was seeing in the hospital daily. It was a difficult time for so many of us, and I believed our entire world was crying out for a solution, for some relief. Maybe I was naive, but the availability of the COVID-19 vaccine signaled so much to me. It was a sign of hope for this horrible crucible our nation seemed to be going through at the time.

So, no, I did not feel like a guinea pig or a sacrificial lamb at that time or even now. I felt empowered, courageous, and proud to be sitting in that chair, offering up my arm to Guyanese-born Dr. Michelle Chester, who administered the shot to me.

I now know that there were many who offered up their bodies to medicine in the past but did not do so willingly. I stand on their shoulders, and I'm grateful for their sacrifices and the opportunity to offer up myself fully informed and willing to serve my community in that way.

A DARK PAST WORTHY OF PRESENT DISTRUST

I appreciate the history shared by African American, Caribbean, and Brazilian peoples. Although our ancestors' paths diverged in different ports, the legacy of the Atlantic Slave Trade and enslaved peoples brought to the Americas from Africa in the sixteenth and seventeenth centuries continue to impact our lives today.

The more I read about the history of medicine during slavery and eighteenth- and early-nineteenth-century America, the more I am convinced that African Americans who distrust both public and private medicine are within their rights to do so. The documented history can be shocking and depressing: slaves were valued for economic profit yet brutally overworked and given poor medical treatment when sick; widespread experimentation by doctors on slave bodies to find cures for diseases and for testing of medical equipment to benefit whites; the robbing of black gravesites to harvest cadavers for medical schools and hospitals. The atrocities stretch from the early days of the Atlantic Slave Trade to the twentieth century with the infamous Tuskegee Experiment and several other injustices.[31] This dark history is not only in the history books; many families have orally passed down their history of mistreatment and abuse by doctors and the health-care system.

LEARNING MY OWN HISTORY

My high school in Jamaica was known for its rigorous curriculum and for producing top graduates who went on to be successful all over the world. While I learned quite a bit of Jamaican history in school, there were some gaps in my education. This is why I admire my brother. He is always learning, reading, finding things out for himself, and inspiring me to do the same.

---

[31] Other experiments include Operation Big Buzz, a 1950s US military field test that dropped over three hundred thousand mosquitoes in Carver, Georgia, a Black town. The test was aimed at testing the feasibility of using the mosquitoes in bioterrorism. There was also Project MK Ultra, a CIA-run program that subjected many young Black boys to psychological tests without the proper consent of their parents. The declassified document from the US Army is available online at: https://www.osti.gov/opennet/servlets/purl/16006843-5BAfk6/16006843.pdf.

Also see: Associated Press, "Black Savannah Residents Haunted by Memory of Mosquito Experiment, *Atlanta Journal Constitution*, February 6, 2021, https://www.ajc.com/news/nation-world/black-savannahians-haunted-by-memory-of-mosquito-experiment/XQKXVGK3MJEHDEMFIDRVRHIPYI/.

The history of plantation medicine in the Caribbean colonies, as in the American South, is a complicated one. While slaveowners had a financial interest in keeping their slaves healthy, sick slaves were indeed used for medical testing, and the bodies of deceased slaves were used for a variety of experiments. Some of these experiments were race-neutral, and other marginalized groups, including indentured workers, sailors, prisoners, the mentally ill, and even children, were used as subjects. I was disheartened to think of what my ancestors endured at the hands of people so indifferent to their humanity.

CARIBBEAN PLANTATION MEDICINE: DOING HARM

Stanford Professor Londa Shiebinger's book *Secret Cures of Slaves: People, Plants, and Medicine in the Eighteenth-Century Atlantic World* chronicles plantation medical experimentation and explores the contributions of enslaved peoples to the medical advances that benefit us today. Shiebinger's work is honest and detailed in profiling the complicated personalities of the doctors who used enslaved people in their research. Following are just three doctors described in Shiebinger's book who used slaves and other disempowered peoples to conduct medical experiments during slavery.

- Colin Chisholm, a British surgeon who worked and lived on the island of Grenada in the late eighteenth and early nineteenth century, conducted several experiments involving Black slaves to determine the basics of core body temperature in different climates and during the spread of a West Indian fever epidemic from 1793 to 1795.[32]
- John Quier, a Jamaican doctor of British descent and slaveowner, practiced medicine in the 1700s and 1800s and experimented on slaves with a smallpox inoculation in 1768.

---

[32] Londa Shiebinger, *Secret Cures of Slaves: People, Plants, and Medicine in the Eighteenth-Century Atlantic World*, Stanford University Press, 2017, p. 35.

- James Thompson, who considered John Quier to be a role model, experimented with slave bodies in the 1810s, including enslaved children, to find an inoculation for yaws, which was a leading cause of disability and severe disfigurement for enslaved people on the islands.

These were powerful, well-respected men, both in their profession and among the plantation owner class. Their methods and practices, beyond the cruelty, defied understanding at times. John Quier, for instance, employed several black assistants in his practice and research work. James Thompson not only conducted experiments on the enslaved; he experimented on poor whites and even himself.

Plantation doctors also sought out enslaved people for their knowledge of traditional cures brought with them across the Atlantic. While these doctors would mostly pretend to ignore and would publicly ridicule the traditional healers and "witch doctors" on the plantations, they sometimes secretly and blatantly stole from them, using African herbal remedies for inoculations against smallpox and yaws, for instance.

Despite their degradation and exploitation, skilled slaves did effectively care for and treat one another with traditional medicines. They did so in spite of laws, like a 1764 ordinance banning "negroes and people of color, free or slave" from practicing medicine in the French colonies. Slaves continued their healing practices on each other. In the 1790s, enslaved doctors and surgeons on the island of Barbados were written about and even praised. Professor Shiebinger describes British military physician George Pinckard praising "Negro doctors" on the island of Barbados and describing Pinckard's surprise at seeing an African slave perform a surgical operation with "greater dexterity" than any top surgeon in Europe.[33]

The established plantation medical system derided most African-derived cures as Obeah or witchcraft, ridiculing these methods as untested and ineffective. Some colonies went as far as to outlaw these practices.

---

[33] Londa Shiebinger, *Secret Cures of Slaves: People, Plants, and Medicine in the Eighteenth-Century Atlantic World*, Stanford University Press, 2017, p. 130.

Interestingly enough, the European doctors grasping about with primitive research methods did not view their own medical experiments as magical. "…[W]hat was diagnosed as "imagination" in Europeans was judged "superstitious" in Africans." [34]

The well-known story of Onesimus, an enslaved man living in 1721 Massachusetts, who introduced Cotton Mather, a doctor and minister, to an effective technique of inoculation against smallpox should encourage all of us. Onesimus was among many enslaved people who, despite his status, contributed to the cures and medical advances we have today.

HOW DO WE MOVE ON FROM OUR COMPLICATED HISTORY?

With this complicated history, I still hold firmly to my conviction on taking the COVID-19 vaccine. I also strongly advocate for people of color to participate in clinical trials and testing. The percentage of Black participants enrolled in new trials for new cancer drugs is alarmingly low, increasing to 3.6 percent from 2.9 percent from 2008 to 2018.[35] The US government has established requirements for broad representation in drug testing, and since 1985, the Federal Drug Administration has required sponsors of new drug applications to show specific data for racial groups and to report demographic data on the trials of investigational new drugs.[36] We, as descendants of slaves, have always had a role in medical advances, willing or not, and are in a much better position today with an entire body of law protecting US citizens from unethical medical practices and giving us the right of informed consent.

Public and private health systems can do more to encourage Black people to participate in clinical trials and research. For one thing, hiring researchers who look like the community they are studying would go a

---

[34] Londa Shiebinger, *Secret Cures of Slaves: People, Plants, and Medicine in the Eighteenth-Century Atlantic World*, Stanford University Press, 2017, p. 126.

[35] Thomas J. Hwang and Otis W. Brawley, "New Federal Incentives for Diversity in Clinical Trials," *New England Journal of Medicine*, 387 (October 13, 2022): 1347–49, https://www.nejm.org/doi/full/10.1056/NEJMp2209043.

[36] Ibid.

long way in building trust. Also, recognizing the unique challenges and limitations of working-class populations would help organizers of clinical trials and research studies tailor these programs to the populations they wish to study. For example, scheduling visits to a medical office in the middle of the workday might not be a viable option for many working people, particularly parents.

Our communities have good reason to be skeptical and to acknowledge our scars from the brutal past of slavery, racism, and exploitation. It takes great resilience and courage to acknowledge this painful past and to trust institutions and systems that have not proven themselves friendly to our communities.

OUR HISTORY IS STILL BEING TOLD

We cannot allow ourselves to remain mired in the past, particularly when our health and our very lives are at risk. Our entire story as a people is still being told. Historians are still discovering how doctors in the eighteenth century benefited from West African healing practices brought to the plantations of the Americas and indigenous cures from the Taínos and other native peoples.

It is difficult to square up the competing realities of the past and present. While we need more people of color involved in testing and clinical trials at every stage for new therapies, we do not want to be taken advantage of because of our ethnicity and comparative lack of power.

How did I do it? Well, as you may have already guessed, I am an optimist, always looking forward. Not in a naive, uninformed way, mind you. My professional and personal experience in health care has shown me the good, bad, and ugly. But I like data, research, and as much information as I can possibly arm myself with. Where I am lacking, my colleagues, my brother, and my friends who know more than me, i.e., people I trust, can fill in the gaps. My hope is that members of our community can develop relationships with trustworthy personal physicians, nurses, social workers, and others who can help us overcome this history of mistrust of medicine.

The ugliness in our past does not have to dictate our future. We can conduct more historical investigation and proudly proclaim and demand credit for our ancestors' contributions to modern medicine. I am not a politician, so I will not try to give a political speech, but I will take this to a personal level. Can we mourn for our ancestors whose bodies were misused and abused by unscrupulous and even evil individuals who sought to benefit economically and professionally off of fellow humans made in the image of God? Can we also honor our ancestors' memory and sacrifice by living the healthiest lives we can? And can we try to process our anger and hurt over the past in a healthy way so we can experience joy and hope for the future?

CHAPTER 26

Taking the Vaccine

"**Y**ou are one person whom the world will remember," UN General Assembly President Abdulla Shahid remarked in a ceremony where I was honored for being the first person in the United States to be vaccinated against the COVID-19 virus. I still have moments of disbelief when I hear these words spoken about me and when I attend events with these highly distinguished people. But if you have read what my staff and I experienced during 2020–2021, I hope you can see that taking the vaccine was something I felt I had to do.

By the summer of 2020, many fortunate people had begun to learn how to live with COVID-19, taking biking and camping trips for their summer vacations instead of traveling abroad. Others were simply stuck at home with their families, but life wasn't all about safe social distancing and outdoor dining. In some regions, the increasing unemployment rate and shutdown of social services began to manifest in negative ways for families and communities. For example, murder rates in eight states increased 40 percent from 2019 to 2020, according to one Pew study.[37]

By the end of 2020, the COVID-19 death toll had reached approximately three hundred thousand people in the United States alone, and officials had no idea whether that number would double in a month, six months, or a year. Public officials were back to considering shutting down schools and businesses. Downtown areas were quiet and deserted as many professionals still worked from home. Many of our essential workers were struggling, grateful for government support but suffering from job losses or massive cutbacks in their work hours. It was high time for vaccines to become a reality.

A TEAM EFFORT

My colleague Dr. Michelle Chester, who administered the vaccine to me, had done valuable work early during the pandemic to benefit our communities. Among her many responsibilities as an executive at Northwell, she worked tirelessly to set up numerous testing sites in communities of color and internally for Northwell employees. In the early summer of 2020, Dr. Chester helped set up numerous testing areas in high-risk communities as part of Northwell's outreach to areas that were being disproportionately hit by COVID-19. Those testing centers served a great need because the public largely was still afraid of leaving their homes and being exposed to the virus. Our organization was key in making COVID-19 tests available to those who desperately needed them.

Several of my colleagues, all doggedly committed to seeing the end of the pandemic, had volunteered to be vaccinated, and they all received the jab that day. I still don't remember how I ended up being the first to sit in that chair. Every one of us in that conference room had been involved in fighting COVID-19 and was committed to stopping its spread. I simply volunteered and was more than ready since I had been waiting for this

---

[37] John Gramlich, "What We Know About the Increase in U.S. Murders in 2020," Pew Research Center, October 27, 2021, https://www.pewresearch.org/short-reads/2021/10/27/what-we-know-about-the-increase-in-u-s-murders-in-2020/.

day for a long time and was excited that it was finally here. I was happy to see my colleague Dr. Yves Duroseau, Vice President emergency medicine for Northwell's western region. Dr. Duroseau, a Black man, is the second person in the U.S. to receive the COVID-19 vaccine.

Although I had no idea that I would hold this prominent place in history I would have gotten vaccinated that day anyway. It was important for me to instill confidence in the public and I feel blessed and grateful to have done this noble act for humanity. I believe now that the decision to vaccinate a critical care nurse, a Black woman, and minority in so many respects was more than fitting.

On December 14, 2020, I walked down to the conference room with an extra pep in my step. I was surprised to see there was a feed on the big screens in the room and I was told that the governor of New York and other state officials would be streaming in. My President and CEO along with other senior leaders and leaders at Northwell and LIJMC, began to fill the room. I was calm, interacting with my colleagues, pacing the room, and anxiously awaiting the vaccine so that I could get back to work. I remember Michael Goldberg, the executive director and Chris Boffa, associate executive director of operations at LIJMC asking if I was okay, constantly checking on me and offered bottles of water while I waited. The wait seemed like forever, after all I was early. There were cameras there, but I was naïve to the magnitude of what was about to happen.

Five of us received the Pfizer vaccine; we all used the same chair. I still chuckle that the Smithsonian has kept the scrubs, my ID, socks, a pair of clogs that had literally fallen off my feet one day, needles, syringe, the vaccine bottle, and everything else from that day in their museum. On that day, it just didn't seem like I was doing anything that important.

Honestly, I wasn't afraid as it happened. I was surrounded mostly by people I knew and had worked with for years, people I trusted. And there was just the common-sense part of it for me. I had taken many vaccinations in the Caribbean with much less medical knowledge than I had currently. I just had no fear. That wasn't a universal feeling. I recall one colleague, Mavis Knox, chief clinical information officer, asking permission to pray over me before I went to take the jab. I let her pray—because I love her, and she's a great person. She is a hard worker who worked tirelessly with my team and I during the pandemic. I believe in God and pray daily. I had prayed that morning for a safe return home like I did every morning during the pandemic.

Still, it all just seemed like another regular vaccination to me. That may have been due to the way I live my life: thankful and ready to do my best every day. I'm not afraid of death, and thankfully, I had no adverse reaction to the vaccine that day or since then.

TRUSTING THE SCIENCE

Yes, it sounds like a cliché now, but I did and still do trust the science.

I had read reports on the evolution of the mRNA technology used to deliver the vaccine internally, which had existed since at least 2009. As a nurse for three decades, I had seen virus outbreaks before, so I knew that scientists, researchers, and the pharmaceutical industry were not completely in the dark about coronaviruses. In 2003, for instance, National Institutes of Health scientists were able to get a SARS vaccine to stage-one clinical trials in twenty months.[38] I was also aware (and in awe) of the unprecedented power, concentrated might, and capability of our nation's research, government, pharmaceutical, and manufacturing best and brightest to bring this vaccine to the American people.

Messaging was a problem for people who already had concerns about vaccines, and confusing coverage in the media may have contributed to some of their doubts and fears. Terms like "warp speed" could have sent the wrong message. Maybe that term failed to communicate the groundwork already laid in developing other vaccines. The messaging could have included more frequent reminders that our public health system had experienced other outbreaks like polio, Ebola, MERS, Zika, and SARS, where rapid activation of vaccine development and public-private

---

[38] Janell Ross, "Working on Coronavirus Vaccine Trials, Kizzmekia Corbett Is 'Not Your Average' Scientist," NBC News, April 12, 2020, https://www.nbcnews.com/news/nbcblk/scientist-kizzmekia-corbett-leads-way-covid-19-vaccine-trials-dedication-n1181626.

health partnerships were initiated. The US was not new to this rodeo. The rhetoric and messaging seemed to have fed fears that the vaccine development was a haphazard process and important safety steps were left out.

What truly disappointed me was the fact that Black people were underrepresented in the clinical trials. One study found that in the Pfizer BioNTech mRNA vaccine study, Black or African Americans represented only 3–9 percent of the participants, and Asians 1–8 percent. In the Moderna phase 1, 2, and 3 clinical trials, White participants accounted for 89–98 percent of the enrollments for the phase 1/2 clinical trial and 79 percent for the phase 3 clinical trial.[39] The virus was killing people of color at the highest rate at one point in the pandemic. But representation of African Americans in the testing trial phase of the vaccine was dismally low. There are many lessons to be learned from the missteps that were made, including how to educate and address people's fears and concerns in a respectful and targeted manner. But overall, I would encourage us to use our agency to get involved in these processes at every step.

While the vaccine debate was over-politicized, we can probably all agree that the rate of deaths steadily slowed once the vaccines were introduced to the wider public. We can probably agree, too, that vaccines in general—measles, polio, influenza—have increased life expectancy and quality of life across the globe. People from marginalized communities are at increased risk of poor outcomes from disease, and we cannot afford to be anything less than vigilant in protecting ourselves, and that means taking full advantage of the protections of vaccination.

---

[39] Lana Khalil et al., "Racial and Ethnic Diversity in SARS-CoV-2 Vaccine Clinical Trials Conducted in the United States," *Vaccines*, 10, no. 2 (February 2002): 290, https://www.ncbi.nlm.nih.gov/pmc/articles/PMC8875029/.

CHAPTER 27

Chronic Disease in Our Communities

I have discussed my grandmother's long struggle with hypertension and diabetes. As a kid, my siblings and I helped give her medications, traveled long distances with her to doctors' appointments, and learned how to cook healthy foods that would not exacerbate her condition. Many of my friends and family today struggle with similar health issues, and I am sure that is the same for you. The CDC reports that six in ten US adults have a chronic disease, and four in ten have two chronic diseases. Indeed, my grandmother lived with two.

Chronic diseases include everything from arthritis, cancer, heart disease, stroke, and lupus, according to the CDC. Common risk factors for these diseases are excessive alcohol use, tobacco use, physical inactivity, and poor nutrition.[40] Chronic diseases are the leading causes of death

---

[40] "Chronic Disease Fact Sheets," National Center for Chronic Disease Prevention and Health Promotion, Centers for Disease Control and Prevention, https://www.cdc.gov/chronicdisease/resources/publications/fact-sheets.htm.

and disability in the US and are leading drivers of the nation's $4.1 trillion in annual health-care costs. Those are scary numbers. Even scarier is that poor, Black, Native American, and other marginalized groups suffer from these diseases at a much higher rate than Whites. In addition to the risk factors I listed above, some researchers believe that Black Americans' risk factors for chronic disease can be partly attributed to the toxic stress from experiencing racism and bias.[41]

WHAT OUR BODIES ARE UP AGAINST

Chronic disease is not the entire story. Where we live, our family background, and our income levels also play a role in our overall health. Here are some very basic examples. For kids with asthma, living in a neighborhood where environmental pollution is prevalent can mean an increase in asthma attacks. Air pollution can cause irritation and trigger asthma attacks. Events such as the water crisis in Flint, Michigan, also show us the harmful effects of living in neglected areas susceptible to pollution. Social problems, like gun violence, fractured families, and mass incarceration, only worsen health outcomes by triggering mental illnesses and instability in families' lives.

What about food security? The lack of access to grocery stores that sell healthy food can leave families with fewer nutritional choices, leading to slower rates of child development and, yes, chronic disease over the long term. Our attitudes toward food, including eating for emotional comfort, eating on the go, and not eating enough nutritious food, all can contribute to sickness in our bodies. A lack of education and misconceptions about fighting disease can also hurt us. For instance, making changes in our diet and daily activity can vastly improve our quality of life. It is a dangerous misconception that healthy food is not fulfilling or tasty. There is much we can learn about food and how to prepare it.

---

[41] Arline T. Geronimus et al., "'Weathering' and Age Patterns of Allostatic Load Scores Among Blacks and Whites in the United States," *American Journal of Public Health*, 96, no. 5 (May 2006): 826–33, https://doi.org/10.2105/AJPH.2004.060749.

As a lower income person living in the Bronx during the 1980s and '90s, I saw many of these problems up close and even experienced some of their effects. My current advocacy position, however, unintentionally reopened my eyes to the overwhelming problems of health inequity our communities face. The fight for our health is not simply a matter of eating right and exercising. The real work begins on a society-wide level, and the solutions involve a multipronged approach. Much like the COVID-19 vaccine effort brought together medicine, research, government, pharmaceutical, and manufacturing sectors, so will the fight against health inequity require partnerships and collaboration across multiple sectors. Still, every one of us can do our part to actively pursue better health for ourselves and our communities.

SOCIAL DETERMINANTS OF HEALTH

The World Health Organization and the CDC share the view that factors other than, say, smoking or a terrible diet can contribute to poor health. The WHO defines the social determinants of health as "the non-medical factors that influence health outcomes." These factors include societal conditions into which people are born and reared and the societal forces and systems that shape their lives, including economic, political, and social systems.[42] These nonmedical factors, of which there are many, can manifest themselves in a lack of access to affordable and quality health care, a lack of proper education, food insecurity, unsafe living conditions, and discrimination.

Dr. Arline T. Geronimus has studied for decades the health impact of enduring oppression and injustice (a concept she describes as "weathering") and found that Black people of all social classes, including those with college degrees and higher incomes, experience poorer health outcomes than all whites.

The social determinants of health may not simply be an American problem borne out of the history of slavery. It is a global problem that

---

[42] "Social Determinants of Health," World Health Organization, https://www.who.int/health-topics/social-determinants-of-health#tab=tab_1.

manifests itself through how climate change affects certain countries, how wars and political conflicts limit access to health care, how relatively cheap tests for diabetes factors remain hard to find in developing countries, and why malaria and viruses like Zika and dengue can disproportionately harm certain populations while wealthier countries can quickly mobilize (and sometimes hoard) vaccinations and treatments.

WHAT ABOUT PERSONAL RESPONSIBILITY?

As humans, we are always looking to identify the simplest answers to our problems, even the most complex ones! If only we could all just eat more fruits and vegetables, exercise forty-five minutes a day, get eight hours of sleep, and get our annual checkups, surely these chronic disease rates would spiral down. But anyone who has lived in the real world knows it's simply not that simple.

Dr. Donald A. Barr, in his widely read book *Health Disparities in the United States: Social Class, Race, Ethnicity, and Health*, lays out a framework showing how low social status can affect a person's health. Dr. Barr posits that when a "person is in a position of low relative status within an established social hierarchy, there are immediate consequences." He argues that a low-social-status person might be more likely to smoke, make poor dietary choices, be physically inactive, and abuse alcohol or drugs. All these activities can lead to cellular and tissue injury and, subsequently, serious disease and/or death. Dr. Barr adds that people with low social status can live in neighborhoods with low social capital, increasing their exposure to environmental toxins and pollutants and psychosocial stressors, both of which can lead to cellular inflammation and damage.[43] These problems do not only affect adults. Dr. Barr writes that economic disadvantage and living in low-social-status neighborhoods have

---

[43] Donald A. Barr, *Health Disparities in the United States: Social Class, Race, Ethnicity, and the Social Determinants of Health, Third Edition*, Johns Hopkins University Press, 2019, p. 96.

profound effects on children's health and how their genetic inheritance is expressed.[44]

Other experts have studied the health-related impacts of racism. A *New York Times* report on Dr. Arline Geronimus's work explained that the concept of weathering calls to mind a rock being steadily worn down because of sustained exposure to rain, snow, wind, and all the elements. It is no wonder that people of color and those with lower socioeconomic status report more severe and more frequent rates of stress.[45] I highly recommend further reading on this idea of how racial stressors can contribute to poor health. Two excellent books that cover the topic are *Under the Skin: The Hidden Toll of Racism on American Lives and on the Health of Our Nation* by Linda Villarosa and *Weathering: The Extraordinary Stress of Ordinary Life in an Unjust Society* by Dr. Arline Geronimus.

I USED TO LIVE THERE!

I can personally attest to much of what Dr. Barr is arguing in his book. Living at the lower rungs of society can lead people to make decisions that seem inevitable in one moment, although the long-term impact on their health is negative. As a new immigrant in the 1980s, I had very little money to spend on healthy foods, and I did not have health insurance. I worked as a cashier at a Bronx supermarket, standing on my feet all day, even when I was several months pregnant. It was a terrible, demoralizing job that paid less than four dollars an hour, which I sometimes supplemented with other work. When I worked at a convenience store in Brooklyn, I took the subway to and from work daily—rain, snow, or shine—like many in my community. The last thing I wanted to do when I got home at night, emotionally and physically exhausted, was go to the gym—not that I could afford a gym membership anyway.

---

[44] Ibid, p. 195.

[45] Alisha Haridasani Gupta, "How 'Weathering' Contributes to Racial Health Disparities," *New York Times*, April 12, 2023, https://www.nytimes.com/2023/04/12/well/live/weathering-health-racism-discrimination.html.

When I became pregnant, I visited the nearest community health center for my prenatal care. It was not comfortable, and I always hated going there. That is one of the barriers to achieving health equity I will discuss in the following chapter. It's bad enough to be poor and sick, but sometimes, the prospect of receiving substandard care from health professionals who come across as uncaring can keep some of the poorest and most in need from even seeking care.

In our sixth-floor walk-up apartment, we ate a lot of rice and carb-rich foods without much thought to a balanced diet. I was eighteen or nineteen at the time and weighed about ninety pounds. I wasn't worried about my weight, so I wasn't too worried about my health. The neighborhoods around Fordham Road in the Bronx, where I lived with my sister and cousin, were teeming with bodegas and fast-food restaurants. The choices for healthy, nutritious food that was also affordable were pretty small. The congested neighborhood was also not conducive to outdoor exercise or calm, stress-free living. There was always something disruptive going on—an ambulance or police car racing by, a traffic incident, firetrucks trying to maneuver through a traffic jam, random neighborhood conflicts. That was just city life. Back then, I wasn't thinking about stress, anxiety, fear of violence, poor nutrition, and the effects on me and my neighbors. I accepted that as life in a big American city.

The people I saw on the BX12 bus or on the subway on my way to work were as hurried and stressed as I was. Those scenes from my early days in the US are a far cry from the scenes I now witness in my Long Island neighborhood, with its manicured lawns, lush green parks, walking trails, and lots of farmers markets overflowing with produce. I find it easy to go for a daily walk now, and it's the highlight of my day. I can choose to grow vegetables in my garden, but the grocery stores in my neighborhood sell all manner of healthy foods with vegan and gluten-free options for everything. It's a contrast I hope will never leave my consciousness as I advocate for those who live in neighborhoods like my former home in the Bronx.

CAST BLAME OR SEEK SOLUTIONS?

Eating right and exercising are not the only determinants of good health, and poor diets and physical inactivity are not the only culprits behind chronic disease, although they certainly do not help anyone on the path to good health. Still, casting blame hardly ever solves anything and can sometimes only further increase health disparities. It was common to hear media pundits blaming people with existing medical conditions for getting infected with COVID-19. For example, people who were obese or who had illnesses linked to poor diets or lack of exercise were ridiculed by comedians and some media figures while they suffered. That kind of cruelty only shows the amount of advocacy and education that is needed about chronic disease and the social determinants of health. There were a great number of people who did not have those diseases who became sick and died from the virus. The fact is, we may never know the full story of why some were infected and some were not and why some died while others survived. But we can do what is within our control to make sure we are not contributing to our own ill health.

CHAPTER 28

Widening Boundaries of Chronic Disease

D uring my first year at the supermarket job in the Bronx, I was still brand new to the United States and still learning about Americans and their way of life and how I needed to adapt. I was always fascinated by the shopping carts people brought to the cash register. There were so many frozen foods, trays of TV dinners, and tons of processed foods like cereals, breakfast bars, cold cuts, and such. At my income level, those foods seemed so expensive! I was also surprised to see people eating and snacking while walking in public, on the subway, or grabbing a large cup of coffee and soda drink on the go. The idea of casual and idle eating was new to me.

THE SIMPLE LIFE

Growing up in Jamaica in the 1970s and '80s, life was much slower, and there were fewer choices when it came to food. Fast food was jerk pan chicken or pork or roasted corn from a roadside vendor. Frozen food maybe ice cream? The idea of heating up leftovers was unthinkable; there would be no such thing in our house anyway. In my grandparents' home, meals were very structured. We had porridge for breakfast before school. Porridge was a form of hot cereal, cornmeal boiled with coconut milk with spices like cinnamon added to it. Yes, brown sugar was added as well. It was a delicious way to start the day that would fill our bellies for the walk to primary school. Until high school, we walked home for lunch, usually fish and root vegetables and a starch, then walked back to school. In the evenings, we had light supper around 6:00 p.m. It was similar to small-town life in a lot of places.

Once I was old enough to buy my own lunch at school, I went for more savory choices and, I'd argue, less healthy. Warm beef patties with coco bread with vanilla or cherry malt or a sky juice or festival or Ovaltine biscuits were my favorites. My classmates and I had our go-to vendors for baked goods; Brother Willie's sky juice with different syrups, which we would mix and match, was legendary. But these were treats, not my main meals.

My grandfather was a farmer who ensured that we had fresh ground provisions delivered to the city, where I would collect the hefty burlap bag of yam, green banana, cocoa, dasheen, and cassava weekly. Many times, I would be the one preparing family meals on the weekends when the helper was off duty once my older sister emigrated to the United States. When we went to the cafeteria for lunch, Ms. Inez's, had our fried chicken breast, rice, and peas, with a salad of shredded cabbage, cucumber, carrot, and tomatoes waiting.

During high school, our neighbor, Ms. Inez, would look out for Garfield and me. Even if we were away from home, we could show up at Ms. Inez's, and our fried chicken breast, rice, and peas, with a salad of shredded cabbage, cucumber, carrot, and tomatoes, would be waiting.

On Saturdays, everyone in the family did chores, cleaning and scrubbing around our property. My siblings and I had our tasks to complete daily or weekly. My job was always to sweep the veranda and driveway and to rearrange the chairs on the veranda. I'll never forget it. Then, in the evenings, we baked rock bun and coconut bread with my grandmother.

On Sundays, we all went to church. Then we had dinner promptly at 2:00 p.m., typically a heavy meal with beans, rice, fish (and meat for the ones who ate meat), and vegetables. Then, we were set free to play. My siblings and I made up our own games and ran around for hours. Around 6 p.m., we would have supper. Then, there were always community sports on a weekly basis.

My grandfather was known in our community for his cola champagne soda with sweetened condensed milk drink. It was served every Sunday evening for supper with whatever we baked on Saturday. This was our last meal before getting ready for the school week and retiring to bed.

We were an active family, but our pace of life was measured and slow. We could literally stop and smell the flowers in our back and front yards. Food was always an event, surrounded by family, activities, and conversations with my siblings, mother, and grandparents. Food was not just a hobby or something one grabbed out of boredom. First, it took a lot of time to prepare it. It took time before a bunch of bananas or plantains made their way from the tree in the backyard to our plates. You had to at least take the time to sit and enjoy the hard work put into it. Food, the growing of it, the sharing of it, the gathering of it, was community, as it has been for cultures around the globe since the beginning.

But the rise of fast food, snacking on the go, and a prevalence of sugary and unhealthy foods is destroying our communities' historically healthy relationship with food and, in some ways, making food our enemy.

JAMAICA'S MODERN SHIFT

The Jamaica Gleaner, the newspaper of record of my island nation, has noted in several reports the unfortunate, increasing rates of chronic disease in the Caribbean. In November 2022, the *Jamaica Gleaner*[46] highlighted a report from the Pan American Health Organization (PAHO), a division of the WHO, that examined the prevalence of diabetes in the Americas region. PAHO's report[47] noted that in recent decades, "the burden of diabetes has increased exponentially, especially in low- and middle-income countries." Heart disease and diabetes took the first and second spots in leading causes of disability-adjusted life years in the Americas region. The number of cases of diabetes is at an all-time high, with a total of sixty-two million people living with the disease, according to PAHO. Also alarming: Two-thirds of adults in the Americas are overweight or obese, and only 60 percent get enough exercise. The report underlined another major health threat: Only twelve countries in the Americas have the six basic technologies required to manage diabetes in their health facilities, including equipment for measuring blood glucose and key testing apparatus.

Jamaica's health and wellness minister has sounded a rallying cry to citizens, calling on them to change their lifestyles. According to the health minister, too many Jamaicans were living with chronic diseases.[48] Some of the statistics cited by Jamaica's health and wellness minister in the *Gleaner* report:

- An estimated 236,000, or 9 percent of Jamaicans, have diabetes, and only 106,000 of these persons, or 45 percent, are aware they have the disease. Additionally, 95,030 have one or more complications related to diabetes.
- Approximately 679,000, or a quarter of all Jamaicans, have hypertension, with only about 54 percent, or 374,000, aware that they have the disease.

---

[46] "PAHO Reports Increase in Diabetes Cases across the Caribbean," *The Gleaner*, November 13, 2022, https://jamaica-gleaner.com/article/caribbean/20221113/paho-reports-increase-diabetes-cases-across-caribbean.

[47] "Panorama of Diabetes in the United States," Pan American Health Organization, 2022, https://iris.paho.org/bitstream/handle/10665.2/56643/9789275126332_eng.pdf?sequence=1&isAllowed=y

[48] "Tufton Sounds Alarm on Lifestyle Diseases," *The Gleaner*, May 4, 2023, https://jamaica-gleaner.com/article/lead-stories/20230504/tufton-sounds-alarm-lifestyle-diseases.

- In 2020, almost 7,500 Jamaicans had a stroke, and 2,400 died from stroke.

THE VIEW FROM THE GROUND

My brother Garfield likes to reminisce about the old days in Jamaica. But he also notices the changes in the Jamaican population. "A lot of the issues that we see in lower income communities in America are starting to become pervasive, like diabetes and certain kinds of cancer," Garfield says. "There was cancer when I was growing up there, but not as much as there is now."

He notes that all the major international fast-food brands now have a presence in Jamaica, and they are very popular places to eat. People aren't cooking at home like they did before, he said. "We can remember growing up in Jamaica going to Kentucky Fried Chicken, like, probably once a month. That was like, you know, a big treat because that wasn't something you did every day."

I was so upset recently when a popular donut chain opened in Jamaica to see the long lines of people waiting to pay good money for these donuts and put these diabetes bombs into their bodies. "Why?" I thought. "We have so many delicious, sweet snacks made with locally grown products that have maybe less than half the sugar and fat than these imported products that I honestly can't describe as food."

Garfield also notes that, in Jamaica, people are not moving as much as they used to. "Everybody's on the Internet, on their phones, at home," he observes. "You see the soccer fields, which, on a Sunday evening, used to be packed with people playing and watching games. But they are grazing grounds for animals now because they're not being used."

Since the 1970s and early '80s, Garfield notes, the island's lifestyle norms have changed, and not for the better.

I have heard the excuse in Jamaica that there is not enough time to cook, that life is faster now, and people are always in a hurry with work, parenting, and school activities. So, like in America, they reach for what is quick and easy. However, I am not convinced that island life is at the same pace as life in America. For some of us, the truth might be hidden in the convenience and ease of fast food, not to mention the addictive sugar and fat in some of these foods. Jamaicans have done and can do better. We have acres of land that can be cultivated and used for farming. We have native fruits and vegetables that can be prepared in ways that are healthier and even more tasty than these imported brands. We can imagine and innovate! There is still time for us to make changes and return to our healthier way of living and eating.

Unfortunately, as a developing country, Jamaica does not have nearly the number of resources available in the United States, United Kingdom, or other richer nations. It is frightening to think of our future health as a country if we continue down the current path.

FAST, UNHEALTHY FOOD

It's not simply about making bad choices in what we eat. Sometimes, it's a lack of knowledge and the influences of culture, among other things. For example, when I left Jamaica and moved to the US, I missed the long family dinners we had back home. I lived vicariously through the Sunday dinner scenes from the movie *Soul Food* and longed to create my own Sunday dinner experiences when I could have my own family and dining table. Meanwhile, I worked hard and ate whatever was easy and accessible. I had no idea at the time that I lived in a food desert and that my food choices were potentially setting me on a path to experiencing chronic disease. It didn't help that I was a skinny girl and constantly being told by strangers and friends that I needed to gain weight. After a while, I almost began to buy into the narrative. Thankfully, over the years, I have learned to make better choices. To this day, I make it a point to eat smart. I enjoy riding my bike to the farmers market and filling my basket with fresh produce, fish, and local offerings as often as possible. I grow vegetables in my own garden, and they taste so much better than anything I've ever bought in a store!

WHAT'S IN OUR CONTROL?

For too many in our communities, the lack of access to affordable, quality, nutritious food has resulted in chronic health issues, including diabetes, obesity, cardiac diseases, and mental health disorders. The stressors of everyday life, socioeconomic conditions, and genetics all contribute to whether a person will suffer from chronic disease, or noncommunicable diseases as they are described by experts. If we're poor, then there are some factors we cannot control—for instance, the overabundance of fast-food restaurants depending on your zip code or the food choices available in the grocery stores or supermarkets (if any) in your neighborhood. In an unsafe neighborhood, residents might rightfully avoid going for a walk or playing outside with the children. Environmental factors, such as pollution, low-quality housing, and unclean water, may be beyond our personal power to change.

The reality is no matter where we live, the odds are stacked against us, whether they are factors under or outside of our control. I have been a vegetarian for decades, but I have still seen my weight creep up despite my active lifestyle. Trust me, I understand that it's a battle to achieve and maintain a healthy diet and active lifestyle in our culture of food as a hobby and sedentary living. But it is a battle worth fighting. I'm sharing all of this with you not necessarily to critique the American lifestyle and idealize an imperfect past. After all, the Jamaica of today more closely resembles America in terms of the food consumed, sedentary lifestyles, and the resulting diseases than it did in the 1970s and '80s.

Therefore, we each must take an active role in managing our health and our family's health by making better lifestyle choices so that we can at least reduce our chances of having our lives shortened or our quality of life stolen by chronic disease. And for the problems that seem out of our control, we have a vote and a voice. We can talk to our community and elected leaders and agitate for change. We must use our voice to get those with the power to listen and respond.

CHAPTER 29

My Experience with Implicit
Bias in Health Care

O ver my thirty years in health care, I have been championed
and inspired by amazing people from all walks of life: patient
care technicians, nursing attendants, EMTs, doctors, nurses,
environmental services personnel, administrators, and executives. Some
I will never forget, like Doreen, who encouraged me to finish my associate degree and become an RN. As an overwhelmed single mother of
a toddler studying and working toward my degree, my nursing school
colleagues inspired me not to give up. Decades later, during the height
of the COVID-19 crisis, my colleagues at Northwell cried and laughed
with me through sixteen-hour days when we could barely distinguish
between day and night. People can be fantastic, and when you're surrounded by the right people, there's nothing you can't do.

It's not just my friends and colleagues. Health-care workers show
up every day in some of the most difficult situations and provide professional care to hurting people. I believe most of us enter the profession with a sense of mission, compelled by an inner drive to see others

become whole and healthy. But we are not perfect, and when we're not at our best, our lesser selves can result in harmful consequences for the people we desire to help.

NOT ALWAYS OUR BEST SELVES

Even the most highly trained professionals can make mistakes out of ignorance or their personal, very human shortcomings. Our institutions also are imperfect. Poor training, embedded societal problems, and organizational deficiencies can go unaddressed for decades, even centuries, resulting in health-care inequities like the kinds that manifested during the pandemic.

I would love to think that I hold no biases and that I am always objective with everyone I encounter, but the human brain simply doesn't function that way. We all have biases—good and bad. Implicit bias[49] impacts everyone, and when it comes to race, ethnicity, and socioeconomic status, implicit bias can have deadly consequences.

Implicit bias is an evolving research area, particularly as it impacts medicine. However, social scientists acknowledge the profound effects that implicit bias has had on health-care outcomes, especially for poor minorities.[50] I'll be the first to say that it can be hurtful when we, as dedicated health-care workers, are criticized for our bedside manner, verbally

---

[49] Scientists quoted in the *New York Times* wrote, "Implicit bias is not about bigotry per se. As new research from our laboratory suggests, implicit bias is grounded in a basic human tendency to divide the social world into groups." — Daniel A. Yudkin and Jay Van Bavel, "The Roots of Implicit Bias," *New York Times*, December 9, 2016, https://www.nytimes.com/2016/12/09/opinion/sunday/the-roots-of-implicit-bias.html.

[50] "Research investigating the role of implicit provider bias on healthcare has had mixed results. While only 33% of vignette-based studies found some impact of implicit bias on outcomes, 89% of the studies using real-world patients found some effect of implicit bias on patient care. This trend raises the question of whether vignette- based studies have different effects on the decision making process compared to real-world studies which may more accurately identify disparities in care and characterize the influence of bias in care." — William J. Hall et al., "Implicit Racial/Ethnic Bias Among Health Care Professionals and Its Influence on Health Care Outcomes: A Systematic Review," *American Journal of Public Health*, 105, no. 12 (December 2015): e60–e76, Section 4.2.6, https://www.ncbi.nlm.nih.gov/pmc/articles/PMC4638275/.

abused by patients, or hear terms like "implicit bias" used to describe our manner of treating patients. But it is an area that contributes to health-care inequity, and we should pay attention to it.

Dr. Donald Barr, whose work I referenced earlier, recognizes that the study of racial bias in health care is highly controversial. The high degree of defensiveness around the topic deeply impacts the studies and research done on whether a person's race or ethnicity affects the way they are treated by their physicians. Barr writes that this topic is freighted with physicians' mistaken belief or fear that they are being or will be accused of being racist. He argues that physicians would do well to understand and differentiate among the forms of racial bias in order to work toward eliminating bias of all types. "It is crucially important for physicians to understand the nature of negative stereotypes and feelings of discomfort that are triggered unconsciously in many circumstances when a white physician who grew up in the United States encounters a patient who is black, Mexican American, or of another racial or ethnic minority."[51]

Those stereotypes are very real for many people. An academic survey of thirty-seven qualifying studies between May 2015 and September 2016 examined the role of implicit bias in disparate health-care outcomes for groups of patients. Thirty-one of the studies found evidence of bias in favor of white or lighter-skinned individuals and against darker-skinned patients among a variety of health-care providers across multiple levels of training and disciplines.[52] In a separate study,[53] researchers focused on experiences of discrimination among breast cancer survivors in the Greater San Francisco Bay Area in a medical setting. The study

---

51 Donald A. Barr, *Health Disparities in the United States: Social Class, Race, Ethnicity, and the Social Determinants of Health, Third Edition*, Johns Hopkins University Press, 2019, p. 259.

52 Ivy W. Maina et al, "A Decade of Studying Implicit Racial/Ethnic Bias in Healthcare Providers Using the Implicit Association Test (IAT)," *Social Science & Medicine*, vol. 199 (February 2018): 219–29, https://pubmed.ncbi.nlm.nih.gov/28532892/.

53 Thu Quach et al., "Experiences and Perceptions of Medical Discrimination Among a Multiethnic Sample of Breast Cancer Patients in the Greater San Francisco Bay Area, California," *American Journal of Public Health*, 102, no. 5 (May 2012):1027-34, https://www.ncbi.nlm.nih.gov/pmc/articles/PMC3483911/.

participants reported experiencing both implicit and explicit discrimination, for instance:

- Some participants reported that health-care providers made assumptions based on their race/ethnicity, education, and immigrant status that compromised their quality of care.
- A Black patient said that she felt doctors limited what they told her because the doctors assumed she lacked enough education to understand them.
- Immigrant participants interviewed felt that they were being treated with less respect because they were perceived as not having a lot of education or were being treated as outsiders because of their immigrant status.
- Other patients felt that poor communication because of language differences caused physicians to ignore them and assume they would not understand what was being said.

MY PERSONAL EXPERIENCE

Some people will tell you that they don't need a university study to tell them that biases and disparities exist in health care. And I would be one of those people—although I highly value the research.

I remember a lot of things from the day in 1989 when I went into labor with my son. For one thing, I was terrified and in unbelievable pain. But what made it a million times worse was my shame and confusion at being treated so horribly the moment I stepped into the emergency room. My pregnancy had been challenging. I had always been small and had struggled to gain weight throughout the entire pregnancy. I was likely undernourished and overall exhausted from working the long shifts at my cashier job at the time. I leaned into my mother as we sat in the back of a taxi on the way to the hospital, praying that I would have a short and easy delivery.

When we arrived, the reception in the emergency room was like walking into a steel door. They sent me home right away. "You're not dilated," the nurse snapped after a quick examination.

So, for the next thirteen and a half hours, I sat around my apartment in pure misery under the troubled glances of my mother. I watched episodes of *The Cosby Show* to try to take my mind off the excruciating pain. I have no idea why this portrayal of the perfect Black family was what I chose to soothe me while I waited for my son to enter this world. There was no sleep for me that night.

As soon as the sun came up, I took my bleary-eyed self out of bed and back into a cab through Fordham Road traffic back to the hospital. This time was no different. I felt like I was disrupting the staff's tea and crumpets. The nurses were so rude and condescending.

"You need to leave. Go walk around and don't come back unless your water breaks and your baby is coming out," one of them ordered.

There I was, tears streaming down my face, holding my belly and walking around the Grand Concourse. My mom and I walked together, with her holding me up and telling me I was going to make it and that everything would turn out okay. I think now of how we may have looked to passersby in that high-traffic area: me, young, skinny, and very pregnant; her, middle-aged, comforting and holding me up.

My water finally broke, and the pain overwhelmed me like a tidal wave. I was heaving and sobbing at that point. My entire body was engulfed in pain. But somehow, we made it back into the hospital, only to find that the elevator was stuck, and no wheelchair was available for me. Oh, the misery of that day. Could things get any worse?

When I finally made it into the labor ward, I was processed quickly and harshly. My mother and my questions were ignored. The rude staff made me feel like an intruder and a burden. As I screamed when the pain became unbearable, one nurse hissed, "When you were out there f-ing, f-ing your boyfriend, you didn't know it was going to be painful?!"

I will never forget the rash treatment, their unkind looks, and the roughness in the manner they prepped me—a sudden splash of water on my skin with no warning, a scraping sound, again with no warning or explanation of what they were even doing to me. I was scared and young, feeling completely powerless and voiceless in that hospital room with these nurses who seemed not to care whether or not I was a human being.

Even then, I suspected that it was because I was poor, unmarried, black, on Medicaid, and an immigrant who lived in the Bronx. They didn't need to treat me with respect. What could I possibly do to them? Who would defend me?

Suddenly, as if in a dream, I felt a warm hand on mine. I opened my eyes and looked into the face of a black woman wearing a white coat—a doctor. Behind her glasses, her eyes were gentle, and her voice confident and soft. She held my hand firmly and said, "Don't mind them. I will take good care of you."

To this day, I wish I knew this doctor's name. She made me feel like a human being that day. I can still see her in my mind's eye, soft face, glasses, just emanating kindness and competence. Her act of seeing me, holding my hand, and speaking kind words did so much for me that painful day. This woman doctor epitomized what a health-care giver should be: professional, respectful, and caring. In that moment, I felt my dignity restored, and my anxiety dissipated both for myself and my baby's safety.

MORE THAN HURT FEELINGS

The trouble with implicit bias, social scientists say, is that by its very nature, it operates unconsciously. Negative biases can cause us to act in negative ways, and we don't have to consciously turn on the bad behavior; it just happens. The nurse who was rude and demeaning to me during my son's birth probably was having a hard day, maybe dealing with serious problems in her life. I will assume those things for her benefit. But what is the result of her bad day? She projected onto me the worst stereotypes about young, black pregnant women. Not only that, but she also implied that I somehow deserved the misery I was experiencing. I wonder how she would have treated me had my skin color been lighter, had I been wearing a wedding ring, had she known that my father was a businessman and former politician, had she known that I came from a privileged upbringing in Jamaica, or had she known that I was educated. My point is that as health-care workers, it should be part of our training to be able to see and treat all patients as human beings worthy of the dignity and respect we would want for ourselves.

In her book *Just Medicine: A Cure for Racial Inequality in American Health Care*, Dayna Bowen Matthew, a civil rights lawyer, argues that a "vast body of social science research" confirms that a patient's race and ethnicity influence physicians' medical conduct and decision-making.[54] And it's not only doctors, Bowen Matthew writes. The research may have ignored the implicit biases of nurses, receptionists, insurers, and administrators.[55] The outcomes of implicit bias include clinical disparities in the treatments given to Black patients with serious diseases.[56] Bowen Matthew writes:[57]

> "…the data overwhelmingly showed that compared to whites, minority patients are less likely to receive appropriate medical treatment for cardiovascular disease, cancer, cerebrovascular disease, renal disease, HIV/AIDs, asthma, diabetes, or pain. Moreover, minorities are more likely to receive inferior rehabilitative, maternal, pediatric, mental health and hospital-based medical services than their white counterparts."

Implicit bias and its studied outcomes are complex problems that affect individuals and families in harmful ways that cannot be ignored.

---

[54] Dayna Bowen Matthew, *Just Medicine. A Cure for Racial Inequality in Healthcare*, New York University Press, 2018, p. 35.
[55] Ibid, p. 37
[56] Ibid, p. 60–1
[57] Ibid, p. 57

A CHARGE AND A CHALLENGE

So, what was the outcome of my birthing experience besides the emotional scarring and a lifelong aversion to that particular hospital? My son, the love of my life, was born at a relatively small but healthy six pounds. I stayed the required (at the time) three days in the hospital and was never happier to see my apartment when I was discharged. I will tell you that it would take an act of God for me to return to that hospital to face the labor and delivery staff again. But the experience did give me a deep empathy and understanding of people who sometimes don't seek the care they need, who deeply mistrust the health-care system, and who feel dismissed and judged by health-care workers.

I wish I could say that the wonderful doctor who stepped in to care for me at the last minute is the norm in the medical profession and that her kindness and professionalism are what lower-income and patients from marginalized groups will always experience. That is certainly my hope, but the research does not bear out that conclusion. In Linda Villarosa's 2018 *New York Times Magazine* article[58] on maternal inequities faced by women of color, the women she interviewed felt similarly dismissed by doctors: their pain was ignored and untreated, they felt silenced, and they were treated in a hostile manner. I definitely was not the first or last woman of color to experience bias in the delivery room.

Stereotyping and implicit bias are shortcuts, and our brains need to make shortcuts at times. As critical care nurses, for instance, we can be busy making decisions and caring for patients, managing staff, and a host of other responsibilities. It may sound callous, but maybe we don't feel there's enough time to consider the person in that bed as more than a patient, a diagnosis, or a set of tasks to complete. This is where the dangers of bias rear their ugly head: when we forget we are dealing with an individual created in the image of God, just like you and just like me. As you have seen in these pages, I have been a patient, a nurse, a student, a

---

[58] Linda Villarosa, "Why America's Black Mothers and Babies Are in a Life-or-Death Crisis," *New York Times Magazine*, April 11, 2018, https://www.nytimes.com/2018/04/11/magazine/black-mothers-babies-death-maternal-mortality.html.

mother, a daughter, a sister, a student, and a friend—just like any patient who is wheeled or walks into a hospital or doctor's office or ICU.

The topic of bias will always cause some of us to throw up our defenses. But I hope we can lay them down, even for a minute, to consider the attitudes and beliefs we bring to work and how those attitudes and beliefs affect our patients. How are we leaving them when we walk away from their bedside? Do they feel respected, cared for, and listened to? Or would they prefer to face illness and death rather than having to face us?

CHAPTER 30

Infant and Maternal Care: Protecting Mothers and Babies

On March 4, 2020, my son's partner gave birth to my grandson, who arrived well before his due date. My grandbaby spent the first four months of his life in the neonatal ICU at the height of the pandemic. To make matters worse, we could not visit him once hospitals suspended visits. My son and his partner were left to observe their newborn being cared for by ICU nurses through laptop and cell phone screens, unable to feed him, touch him, or even hear him cry in person.

I struggled to find the words to comfort my son. We had been through so much together as a family. And this was yet another trial I wished I knew how to protect him from. But there was nothing I could do. We simply had to wait for my grandson to become strong enough to be sent home.

My son, who is normally very stoic, broke down in tears at one point from the weight of all the stress and anxiety. It was one of my lowest points as a mother, just feeling so helpless in the face of my child's suffering at what should have been one of his most joyful moments. I wanted to carry that weight for him so badly. I wanted my grandson to be better, at home and safe with his parents, but there was nothing I could do but pray. I could not take away my son's fear and worry. As his mother and with my life experience, I felt I could shoulder his burden much more easily than he could. Instead, I could only walk beside him through the pain.

With the world careening from COVID-19 in the background, the statistics on the Black infant mortality rate kept me up at night. Would this vulnerable little baby be okay in this dangerous environment?

I had to put on a brave face for my son and his partner. They were completely overwhelmed. While most families were hunkered down and hiding from COVID-19, they were traveling back and forth to the hospital to get a few moments with their baby. By the end of the second week, hospital visits ended. Then, forced to stay home, they were watching their baby in the ICU through an iPad screen. We were fortunate because my grandson did pull through and was sent home much healthier, and today, he is a healthy boy full of energy and intelligence. But for a lot of families, the ending is not as happy.

THE BAD NEWS ON BLACK INFANT MORTALITY

In 2016, infants born to black mothers died at the rate of 11.1 per 1,000 births compared to 4.9 deaths per 1,000 for infants born to White mothers. This was in 2016, not 1916! Dr. Donald Barr, in his seminal book, *Health Disparities in the United States: Social Class, Race, Ethnicity, and the Social Determinants of Health*, attributes this gap in infant mortality to a number of factors, among them the higher frequency of black mothers having underweight or low birthweight babies. Chronic disease can play a role. Mothers who have high blood pressure face increased health risks during pregnancy, but so do their babies. Dr. Arline Geronimus writes that "weathering stressors," such as hypertension, high blood pressure, heart disease, and psychological stress, can expose a fetus to negative outcomes. These chronic ailments and stressors can deprive a fetus of nutrients and oxygen and expose the fetus to the impacts of stress response while in its mother's womb.[59]

These health risks follow children from the womb to our communities. Dr. Barr writes that children born into low-income homes and communities can experience "toxic levels of stress" that can lead to poor health outcomes from a young age. He notes that Black and minority families tend to be segregated into neighborhoods with higher levels of air pollution, allergens, and a proliferation of fast-food outlets with few choices for healthy food.[60] "It is essential that we appreciate the profound effects the stress of inequality can have on the development of children."

INEQUITIES IN BLACK MATERNAL HEALTH

In 2022, Northwell Health launched the Center for Maternal Health,[61] a "high-tech, high-touch campaign to reduce the country's maternal mortality rate—the highest among the world's industrialized nations." The center also addresses health risks facing Black women in America, "who are three times more likely to die from pregnancy-related causes than whites." I've had many conversations with the brilliant doctors involved with the center, and I am excited and confident that it will continue to live up to its promise. Improving maternal health is an issue near and dear to my heart. I hope that sharing my experience giving birth as a young, single mother lacking in resources and social capital opened your eyes to some of these problems.

---

[59]   Arline T. Geronimus, *Weathering: The Extraordinary Stress of Ordinary Life in an Unjust Society*, Little Brown Spark, p. 97–8.

[60]   Donald A. Barr, *Health Disparities in the United States: Social Class, Race, Ethnicity, and the Social Determinants of Health, Third Edition*, Johns Hopkins University Press, 2019, p. 195.

[61]   Lisa Barr, "Northwell Announces Center for Maternal Health," Northwell Health, April 5, 2022, https://www.northwell.edu/news/the-latest/northwell-announces-center-for-maternal-health.

Back then, I had no idea that inequities in maternal health were such a widespread phenomenon. I was just a young mother-to-be trying to find the best care for myself and my baby. Thirty-plus years later, there is no denying that this is a systemic issue that, thankfully, is being addressed by the government and the health-care industry. Linda Villarosa's 2018 *New York Times Magazine* article[62] on inequities in maternal health and disparate outcomes Black mothers face sparked much-needed public conversation and prompted an initiative in the state of New York to address maternal mortality and reduce racial disparities in health outcomes, including a pilot program to provide Medicaid coverage for doula services.[63] Villarosa's book *Under the Skin: The Hidden Toll of Racism on American Lives and on the Health of Our Nation* examines even more deeply these problems faced by women of color during their pregnancies and at the point of birth. But I have to warn you: this is heartbreaking information to digest. Villarosa notes that the problem of maternal mortality in the US was worse in 2018 than it was in the previous twenty-five years and that the rate of pregnancy-related deaths for Black women in the United States is higher than the rate for women in poorer countries, such as Mexico.

These are alarming facts that we cannot sweep away. The fact is, for many women of color—rich and poor—it is difficult to bring a baby into this world. Health conditions that existed before pregnancy, illnesses that develop during and after, and, unfortunately, race all play a role in how a woman will experience pregnancy in our nation.

THE DISMAL STATISTICS

- Black women are over three times more likely to die from pregnancy than women from other ethnic groups. According to

---

[62] Linda Villarosa, "Why America's Black Mothers and Babies Are in a Life-or-Death Crisis," *New York Times Magazine*, April 11, 2018, https://www.nytimes.com/2018/04/11/magazine/black-mothers-babies-death-maternal-mortality.html.

[63] "New York State Doula Pilot Program," New York State Department of Health, https://www.health.ny.gov/health_care/medicaid/redesign/doulapilot/.

the CDC,[64] Black and American Indian/Alaska Native women experienced a higher ratio of pregnancy-related deaths (40.8 and 29.7 per 100,000 respectively) than did all other racial/ethnic groups from 2007 to 2016. This pregnancy-related mortality ratio (PRMR) for Black and Native women aged thirty years or older was approximately four to five times that for their white counterparts.

- The disparity regarding race is even greater when you look only at ethnic groups. Even black women at higher income levels are at greater risk for death from pregnancy than women of other ethnic groups in lower income groups. The CDC reports that pregnancy-related deaths among Black women with a completed college education or higher were 1.6 times that of white women with less than a high school diploma. Among all women with a college education or higher, the rate of pregnancy-related deaths for black women was 5.2 times that of their white counterparts.

- Black women face higher rates of preeclampsia (high blood pressure and liver or kidney damage that occur in pregnant women), which puts both the mother and baby at increased risk, and higher rates of Caesarian sections.

- Preexisting conditions, such as chronic disease, lack of access to proper care, and systemic bias, contribute to pregnancy-related deaths. The CDC reports that cardiac diseases and hypertensive disorders contributed to a significantly higher proportion of pregnancy-related deaths among black women than among white women.

MY PREGNANCY EXPERIENCE

It can be heartbreaking as a parent to want to give your child the very best care available but to be blocked at every turn by forces beyond your

---

[64] Emily E. Petersen et al., "Racial/Ethnic Disparities in Pregnancy-Related Deaths — United States, 2007–2016," *Morbidity and Mortality Weekly Report*, 68, no. 35 (September 6, 2019): 762–65, https://www.cdc.gov/mmwr/volumes/68/wr/mm6835a3.htm.

control. When I was pregnant with my son in the 1990s, I felt so isolated and alone up against a foreign health-care system. There I was, at the bottom of the socioeconomic order in New York City, pregnant, unmarried, and a Medicaid patient. At the neighborhood clinics where I got my checkups, good care was elusive. I never saw the same doctor more than twice. By the time I took the bus and subway and waited in the long line for the doctor on duty, it would be an almost daylong affair. I would always have to miss work to make these appointments, and missing work meant a smaller paycheck. I was among the crowds of elderly folks, young pregnant girls, moms with sick toddlers, or adult children with their elderly relatives. Don't get me wrong, I have the utmost respect for doctors, nurses, and staff at neighborhood health-care centers because they meet such a pressing need. The waiting area could be loud and unruly. Someone could crack a joke out of nowhere, sending everyone laughing. A patient could lose their temper and verbally attack the staff. The clinic was worlds away from the pastel-dipped doctor's office visits one gets with BlueCross BlueShield or the concierge health-care services available to high-earning professionals. These health-care centers could be high-stress environments. And for low-income women, like I was at the time, that may be the main source of their prenatal care. I was still lucky compared to other women within my demographic, however. My son was born healthy and thriving despite my negative birth experience.

THIS PROBLEM CAN BE SOLVED

Nearly half of severe maternal morbidity events and maternal deaths are preventable, and improving the quality of health care before and after a woman gives birth may be critical to better outcomes for Black mothers.[65] The CDC has increased awareness around maternal health inequities in recent years and provides wonderful educational resources

---

[65]   Elizabeth A. Howell, "Reducing Disparities in Severe Maternal Morbidity and Mortality," *Clinical Obstetrics and Gynecology*, 61, no. 2 (June 2018): 387–99, https://journals.lww.com/clinicalobgyn/abstract/2018/06000/reducing_disparities_in_severe_maternal_morbidity.22.aspx.

for individuals, communities, and the health-care industry.[66] What can women do to advocate for themselves? The CDC urges women and their families to speak out: talk to a health-care provider if anything doesn't feel right, seek immediate care when experiencing urgent maternal warning signs, and connect with social support systems before, during, and after pregnancy. As women, we must be our own best advocates. Even if we are being treated unfairly, we must speak up for ourselves. Early in the pregnancy, we must seek out doctors and nurses who listen to and care about us. We might need to get a doula involved if that is what makes us feel safe.

Northwell's Center for Maternal Health was launched with the hope of combating inequities in outcomes for Black mothers and infants. Already, there have been signs of progress. The Maternal Outcomes and Morbidity Collaborative (MOMS Program) has already recorded improvement for Black women who enrolled before giving birth. Patients who were monitored by the program were found to have more than 70 percent lower rates of maternal morbidity and readmission to the hospital aafter being part of the Program. More programs like Northwell's Center for Maternal Health, which actively engages marginalized communities and makes women of color feel heard, seen, and cared for, would go a long way in improving outcomes for Black mothers and babies across the country.

---

[66] "Working Together to Reduce Black Maternal Mortality," Centers for Disease Control and Prevention, April 3, 2023, https://www.cdc.gov/healthequity/features/maternal-mortality/index.html.

CHAPTER 31

Strong and Vulnerable: Carrying the Burden of Racism

"The myth of Black women's strength is dangerously seductive in that it imbues Black women with a certain moral and emotional superiority, providing a psychic balm against the daily insults incurred from social injustice. No matter what her lot in life, a Black woman can take comfort in the fact that she is strong, that she possesses the emotional and spiritual fortitude that have enabled her foremothers to withstand suffering and that will enable her to do likewise."

—Too Heavy a Yoke: Black Women and the Burden of Strength by Chanequa Walker-Barnes

"You're the strongest woman I know," Garfield said to me recently. We were reflecting on the past, sorting through memories of the ups and downs and the challenges we've overcome in our lives. I appreciate my brother's compliment; he is not the only person who has described me that way. And if you're a certain type of woman reading this, you might have gotten the same compliment: You're so strong. You're a survivor, a warrior, an overcomer. A boss, shot caller, boss-babe, boss-bitch, or whatever they are calling it these days.

When I read media reports about me, it can be dizzying the way they list my professional journey: From the Borough of Manhattan Community College to a doctorate in health sciences and health-care executive, all achieved as a working, single mother. You should be so proud, I often hear. You did it!

In my immigrant community, it was common to hear that America is not a place to come and sit down and twiddle your thumbs. You have to work hard and do whatever it takes to make it. Once you got that first job, you started thinking about the next one up the ladder. Once you got the bachelor's degree, you began to think about the master's or the PhD. The exhaustion, the sleepless nights, the strained relationships, and the anxiety that came along with this upward mobility were hardly discussed as a negative; it was all just a necessary part of the deal.

If someone had asked me thirty years ago: Why all of this education? Why the relentless drive? The answer would have been: Why in the world not? My father was a high-achieving businessman, politician, and community leader. My grandmother was an educator, and I had seen the difference that education made in my family. Education lifted me out of poverty in America and slowly but surely afforded me a better life and better opportunities for my son. So, yes. It was like discovering a secret. Oh, you mean getting the best education possible is what it takes? Then, I'm on board!

When I had my son, the need to advance became even more critical. The disdain and dismissal that I experienced as a Black immigrant and low-wage worker would never be his experience if I had anything to do with it. What really encourages me is when my son says, "I really admire you, mom. I'm so proud of you. I don't know how you do it with all these degrees and accomplishments." He comes to my graduations and events and cheers me on at every turn. I want him to know that if I can do it, then he can accomplish anything he wants.

Hard work became very familiar to me at a young age; it wasn't new or foreign. I had seen my mother, aunts, and other women in my community do the same thing: power through, pick yourself up when you fall and then start all over again. What could possibly be wrong with that?

JOHN HENRYISM AND BLACK WOMEN'S HEALTH

You may have heard the term John Henryism used to describe the lived experience of Black individuals who spend themselves achieving success to defy stereotypes and negative racial perceptions. The John Henryism Scale of Active Coping is a psychometric test that includes questions that one could say measure a person's grit and determination. John Henryism was coined in the 1970s by Black epidemiologist Dr. Sherman James, based on a folklore character, John Henry, the "steel driving man" who worked himself to death. Dr. Sherman James dedicated an entire body of work to studying the health costs associated with achieving success while contending with racial discrimination.[67] Other researchers[68] have explored John Henryism as it relates to Black women and termed it the "superwoman schema," a reflection of Black women's ability to be "resilient despite great social adversity." This schema, described by social scientist Amanda Perez, can show itself in several ways, including:

(1) feeling an obligation to present an image of strength (even when one doesn't feel strong).

---

[67] "John Henryism," Center for Family Research, University of Georgia, https://cfr.uga.edu/for-researchers/research-digests/john-henryism/.

[68] Amanda D. Perez et al., "Superwoman Schema and John Henryism among African American Women: An Intersectional Perspective on Coping with Racism," *Social Science and Medicine*, vol. 316, 115070 (January 2023), https://www.sciencedirect.com/science/article/pii/S0277953622003768.

(2) feeling an obligation to suppress emotions.

(3) resistance to being vulnerable and dependent on others.

(4) having an intense motivation to succeed (despite limited resources).

(5) feeling an obligation to help others.

This "superwoman schema" can be both a burden and blessing that helps Black women withstand the stress of discrimination but also increases their risk for stress-related diseases, according to Perez. She is not alone in this line of thinking. Dr. Chanequa Walker-Barnes, in her book *Too Heavy a Yoke: Black Women and the Burden of Strength*, writes that the "mythological strength of Black women often masks the very real vulnerabilities of their lives." Dr. Arline Geronimus's work on the concept of "weathering" also renders this phenomenon a threat to health for Black men and women in America. Battling back the stereotypes, hostilities, and discriminatory behavior can have serious physical effects on our bodies. "…[S]uccess comes at a spectacularly high health cost for those who have to fight the hardest to achieve it in the context of a society that doesn't value them."

Indeed, the high rates of chronic disease and related deaths among Black women show that we may not be as strong as we think, and admitting our vulnerability can be one of the healthiest—and strongest—things we can do. Even before COVID-19, Black women were experiencing epidemic rates of stroke and heart disease[69] due to the increased prevalence of risk factors such as obesity, diabetes, hypertension, socioeconomic factors, and stressors such as prioritizing care for others over oneself.

FEELING MY RACE

In earlier chapters, I shared humiliating experiences during the birth of my son and with employers who intentionally withheld wages from me.

---

[69] "African American Women Need to Take Their Hearts to Heart," Mayo Clinic Health System, June 20, 2022, https://www.mayoclinichealthsystem.org/hometown-health/speaking-of-health/african-american-women-heart-health.

But there have been many more experiences that have enraged, shamed, and terrified me. Being a Black woman in America is not for the faint of heart, and we must acknowledge the difficulties that we face and continually seek healing for these racial injuries.

I was fortunate to have a relatively advantaged upbringing, but emigrating to the United States instantly changed my social status. It's not often discussed that Black immigrants can sometimes come to America having never experienced their race as a Black person in a majority white culture. Although Jamaica was poor in relation to the United States, I did have a strong sense of myself as an individual and as a descendant of slaves. But I'd never had to live my life under the constant gaze of a majority culture that sometimes saw me in the most negative light simply because of my skin color. It took a while to accept that, in America, people may attribute certain characteristics, behaviors, and attitudes to me without even knowing where I was from or what I had done in life. In some ways, it felt like the skin I was in told my life story before I'd even had a chance to open my mouth. It was angering, depressing, and frustrating that this was the reality of life in America.

Over the years, I have had to withstand the stress of racism. I have had to have the conversation with myself at work: Am I being mistreated because of my race or for some other reason? When I receive poor treatment in a hotel or a store, it's the same suspicion that I either have to quiet within or address head-on with the person in front of me. It can be exhausting at times.

Even the most mundane life experiences can turn into racial moments. As I have mentioned, I am passionate about gardening. Once, my best friend Pauline and I were shopping for plants. A white well-dressed middle aged woman came up to us. "You're buying a lot!" she said. "Where are you going to plant all of those flowers?" We looked at her in confusion. Then it dawned on me. She may be thinking we are apartment dwellers from the city and couldn't possibly have a yard to plant these blooms. My more sarcastic self wanted to snap back at her. Pauline said I should have told her: "I'm going to put them on my fire escape." Instead, we just ignored her and kept shopping. But this was so frustrating. The way I saw it, my friend and I were two Black girls in this predominantly white neighborhood at this exclusive, upscale nursery buying all these plants. To this woman, there had to be something off. We were not gardeners or landscapers, so what were we? Why couldn't we just be assumed to be like any other customer at the garden center? Pauline and I did have a good laugh on the way home, though. Our car was full, from the back seat to the trunk, with plants, and it really was hilarious to think of where we would put them if we still lived in tiny New York apartments.

This constant internal negotiation, suspicion, and self-questioning can cause many people to lose sleep. It causes the kind of stress that releases cortisol into our bloodstream and starts a chain of negative physiological effects. An incident at work, a store, or a restaurant can release our fight-or-flight hormones. Over years, over decades, how does that impact our health? How does that play into my mental and physical health and how I function as a professional?

I have tried to train myself over the years to quickly get over these thoughts and move on. And I have long been an advocate for daily meditation and prayer. Trust me, it makes a difference. It took so long for me to achieve my goals and find my voice and confidence in this very competitive country. Why would I let a store clerk's ignorance or thoughtlessness ruin my day? There is a time to correct people who are being rude or racist to you. There is a time to walk away, and there's a time to fight; we have to choose wisely. There is a biblical proverb that advises (paraphrased): Do not answer a fool according to his folly, or you yourself will be just like him (Proverbs 26 4:5). I may not always get this right, but as I have gotten older, I am learning to choose me first: my peace, my joy. Getting into arguments with ignorant people about their ignorance is not my idea of time well spent. It's not that racism is not worth fighting. I believe all people have a responsibility to fight racism. For some, fighting verbally and loudly is the way we feel healthy. For others, retreating and meditating is how we retain our peace and sanity. Know yourself and act in your own best interests.

That incident, among many others, reminded me that how I am perceived in America as a Black woman can be far removed from the sum total of my history and life experiences. People who are content to view me through a certain lens, whether out of laziness, ignorance, or hate, might never take the time to know my story but instead will place me in a box, a convenient yet false narrative. It really is up to me to be firm and secure in who I am. I remind myself daily to never live a lie and to embrace my entire self unashamedly. So, here I am, a Jamaican American with a full and complex story that makes up the sum total of me.

NOT ONLY BLACK WOMEN

My brother Garfield is a happy-go-lucky guy, big on owning your own mistakes and taking personal responsibility. But when it comes to being a Black man in America, he will be the first to admit that there's so much that is out of his control.

America has been a long adjustment, he says. In his early years in New York, it didn't bother him when he would be followed around in high-end stores. "I didn't grow up experiencing stuff like that," Garfield says. "So, for me, it was like, if they wanna follow, then follow, you know? That was my thing then." But over time, the overt discrimination became too much to accept, particularly in the workplace. "I was being passed up for promotions or raises, even though I was performing much better than other personnel. That's what was bothering me more than anything else."

Garfield has a doctorate in global health and has written a dissertation on telemedicine. Sometimes he has to remind himself that he is seen as a potential suspect when he leaves his home. Because he has been pulled over in his very nice car, he still seizes up with fear if a police car follows behind him for too long. At the end of the day, you just have to pray, Garfield says. "Every time you see an incident on the news of another brother killed by a cop, you think it could have been you." It's a tough way to face life, he says. "It's just a matter of encountering the wrong person at the wrong time. So, you know, you try to be prepared, but at the end of the day, it's not something that you can truly prepare for. So I think 90 percent of it is just prayer."

Garfield recalls being new to America and starting his first job as an accountant at a real estate firm. "It was shocking to me the differences being an accountant here and being an employee in Jamaica with the racial issues, the way you were treated compared to your Caucasian counterparts."

Being passed over for opportunities and feeling unappreciated for his work made him uncomfortable in the corporate environment. My brother decided to give up on corporate America and went back to school, hoping to do something that would give him more autonomy. Garfield has been a respiratory therapist for over two decades. He has made a conscious effort to avoid certain types of professions because he did not want to have to encounter bias and prejudice in the workplace.

"As a Black man, I think we are probably more stressed than every other category in the society," Garfield says. "Because it's an added burden to always be looking over your shoulder, to always feel like if you ever happen to come in contact with some law enforcement officer. The outcome is probably not gonna be good. And it's something that I live with, and I'm sure, you know, every other Black person, especially men, live with as well."

WEATHERING AND STRESS

Racism and the effects of racism do impact people's health. I not only deal with the stress of personal encounters, but I also carry the weight of worry for my brother, my son, and my grandson. We have been socialized to swallow our emotions. But being constantly triggered by additional incidents of bias can only add to our already heavy burdens.

I had an encounter in my neighborhood during COVID-19 where my white friend, a fellow nurse, and I had a rare weekend day off, and we went out for a drive to get out of the house. On our way back, as I was about to turn to head home, the police appeared, redirecting us to make a U-turn. I was less than a mile from home and so used to driving that way home that I lost my bearings temporarily. I saw a driver ahead of me take a turn I knew could lead to my house. So, I thought I'd ask the officer whether I could make the same turn. But he was so angry and so rough in the way he answered. His attitude even scared my friend. Shaken up, I turned around, collected my thoughts and emotions, and figured out a detour to my house on my own. I was shaken up for days. It really bothered me, and I'm convinced that my skin color had something to do with his nasty attitude. But am I 100 percent sure? No. That uncertainty adds to the stress of it. I never know why I am being treated a certain way, and my antennae must constantly be up so I can quickly move to safety or remove myself from a potentially harmful situation.

We can also face stress from the fear of violence within our own communities. Gang violence and drug-related violence are very real threats that can impact our emotional and physical health. Living in a community where gunshots echo in the night can raise our stress levels. No one should ever have to get used to that.

In Jamaica, the level of crime and violence has risen to unprecedented highs. It pains me to read news reports on the incidents of domestic violence, kids being murdered or being preyed on at such young ages, and several other horrific acts. I often wonder about how younger people are dealing with the violence in their communities and how they will be affected as they grow older.

Gun violence, whether from mass shootings or gang violence, can strike fear in our hearts and cause us to be cautious or mistrustful of strangers or even our neighbors. Our world can seem more dangerous by the day.

Some of us are immobilized by the trauma. We can probably all think of someone we know who is terrified of going to a job interview because of past racial harassment at a previous job, even years ago. Or a person who refuses to drive in a certain part of town, although it has been decades since that part of town was a majority-white district that terrorized people of color. Those emotions take up dwelling space in our bodies and our consciousness, and it takes hefty body, mind, and soul work to dredge them up and throw them away for good.

Many of us in corporate or other professional environments are under constant stress from demanding jobs. We may also face internal and external pressure to prove ourselves at work, to defy racial stereotypes and negative comments regarding having benefited from affirmative action, and face constant heightened scrutiny of our work, of our very own legitimacy. We may be targeted by law enforcement and by our own neighbors in our own neighborhoods simply for being Black. These are difficult realities to navigate life with on a daily basis. Over time, these stressors wear us down and negatively impact our health. And, for some of us, the success we should begin to prioritize might be our health and not our careers or education.

Part of the despair I experienced during COVID-19 was seeing the loss of so many people of color from all social strata. I feared that all of us, including myself, would eventually die from the virus. We are still here, thank God. Still, there are so many other diseases that are killing us slowly—some we can act on and others beyond our control.

We are not entirely helpless because of where we can (or cannot) afford to live, our social and economic status, and the color of our skin. Solutions might involve health policy and political and social action. But we can start on the personal level by becoming advocates against chronic diseases by raising awareness and caring better for ourselves, our families, our neighbors, and our communities.

CHAPTER 32

I'm Not Your Superwoman: Burning the Cape

I enjoy spending time with young people. Their perspective on life can be so different from mine, so I'm always learning from them. For example, some of the younger nurses are much more dedicated to and in tune with their mental health than I ever was in my thirties. They have no problem taking time off from work when life gets too stressful. For me, that was unheard of because stress was just a part of life. I can't say I am on board with all of their ideas and views about life, but they are teaching me a lot and broadening my worldview.

One young woman in her twenties I interviewed for this book had some interesting thoughts on this idea of the Black superwoman who works very hard, cares for her family, supports the community, and does everything else in between. She was not impressed with the idea of the traditional "strong Black woman." She is a recent college graduate considering law school. Her parents are hard-working and raised her in a God-fearing household in a large Northeast city. She has seen plenty of successful Black women doing the superwoman thing, as she calls it. They are not role models for her.

"I feel that some Black women tend to wear a cape and try to save everybody. At the same time, not everyone looks out for Black women or acts in their interest."

When asked whether I should have been the first to take the vaccine, she said she did not think it was necessarily the best decision. Why did it have to be a Black woman? she asked. She believes that my being the first to take the vaccine is another example of Black women being counted on to be everyone's savior.

She says it is the same phenomenon in politics when presidential candidates court Black women to gain the presidency. Black women consistently vote for the Democratic Party candidate in overwhelming numbers.[70] She and other young women see this sort of heroism not as a badge of honor but as a burden. She does not believe that it has helped Black women to be cape-wearing heroes and wants something different for her generation.

"I would not wear the cape because I have seen how it affects women of all generations and ages. I wouldn't try to be the savior when I see the treatment of Black women."

She cites examples such as Serena Williams's struggle in childbirth and the fact that a wealthy Black woman could not escape these poor health outcomes. She's been long bothered by how Serena Williams has been criticized and mistreated by tennis fans and the media, even though Williams is one of the greatest athletes in history. She also believes that Black women are not respected and prioritized in romantic relationships and cites online abusive language toward Black women from men of all races. She felt betrayed when Black women who called out abuse or mistreatment by male celebrities were not believed by others in the Black community. "Even though we are out there advocating and marching for

---

[70]   Megan Botel, "How Black Women Worked to Secure Joe Biden's Election as President," *USA Today*, December 6, 2020, https://www.usatoday.com/story/opinion/2020/12/02/how-black-women-organized-voters-secure-joe-bidens-victory-column/6475054002/.

justice all the time, I feel that we don't get the same support in return," she said.

What is the solution, then? I asked her. She thinks Black women should spend more time prioritizing themselves first, what they want out of life, and not what the community or their families want. "I know that not all Black women wear the cape, but for the ones that do, I wish they would evaluate why they are living their lives in that way. Maybe they should consider burning the cape."

I asked her what "burning the cape" would mean in practical terms. She laughed. "Burning the cape means putting yourself first and not trying to be everyone's savior."

WHOSE HERO?

"Anyone who thinks women who work hard every day just to be called a hero or superwoman is kidding themselves," S.D. says. She is a busy nurse practitioner who has run her own business, sent two children to college, and now takes care of her mother-in-law while working full-time. "I don't see myself as a superwoman, but there were times in my life when I was working too hard until I was forced to slow down," she admitted. "But to me, that's just supporting people I love. That's not wearing a cape."

Her life is less hectic now. She's in her fifties and can take better care of her health and spend more time on the things she enjoys. "But when my kids were younger and things were tight financially, I didn't have a choice. I had to go get that master's degree so that I could earn a higher income. I wasn't satisfied with my kids not having certain opportunities. I wanted each of my kids to have their own room and a house with a yard, and I wanted to pay for their college so they wouldn't have to work. Those are things that I sacrificed for, and I don't regret it."

She also is an immigrant woman of color who has experienced discrimination in America. "My family doesn't have the generational wealth in America. That would probably have made my path a little easier, but those are the breaks. I'm proud of what I've done for my family, and I am proud of my kids and happy that they had a comfortable upbringing. Most of all, it's nice to be able to slow down now in my mid-fifties and focus on me!"

HINDSIGHT IS 20/20

I agree 100 percent. I, too, am finally at a point in life where I can reflect and ask if I would do things differently knowing what I know now. When I look at the man my son has become, my precious grandson, and having my mom with me to enjoy our home together, it's honestly hard to say that I regret anything. But would I do it now, meaning the multiple jobs while going to school to earn multiple degrees? Maybe not.

Don't get me wrong: I believe in working hard and achieving goals. But at the same time, we cannot neglect our mental and emotional health to meet some impossible standard that other people have set for us or that we even set for ourselves.

For example, my son is a happy and well-adjusted young man. He went to college but didn't feel the need to pursue the career path I wanted for him. He is quite productive and content without feeling compelled to earn an advanced degree or become a Wall Street titan or a famous doctor. He's doing great, taking care of his family and being a good father. I ask myself now why I was so worried and stressed about his future. Everything turned out just fine! It may sound cliché, but what mattered most were the times we spent together as a family and the security I could provide by being there for him. So, maybe I could have done a little less work and stopped to smell the roses a bit more often if I knew then what I know now.

***

Being black, a nurse, and now a public figure, that Black superwoman label tends to follow me around, wanted or unwanted. Sometimes just thinking about it can cause feelings of anxiety. When people ask how I'm dealing with my new life as a public figure, I respond that I don't see myself as a celebrity. I don't put undue pressure on myself in that regard. I still wear sweatpants and sneakers and throw on a hat to go to Target or CVS. There's nobody camping outside my door waiting to snap my picture. On a typical Saturday, you'll catch me wearing a silk headscarf, mules, and jeans on my way to a friend's music performance or to meet a girlfriend for dinner. Or you might catch me on a plane, reading and preparing for my next podcast, something I very much enjoy doing.

Self-care is very important to me. I plan for it like it's a job! Some days, when I should be doing something, I choose to just lay on the sofa and watch TV, read a novel, or sleep instead. I try to be thoughtful and recognize when to stop, when to pull back, and when I can extend myself. I've learned to filter some of the speaking and appearance requests that involve a long plane ride. Traveling domestically or internationally can be very hard on the body.

Laura Vanderkam's book, *Off the Clock: Feel Less Busy While Getting More Done*, helped me visualize a more intentional way of planning how to spend my time. Vanderkam does a great job of sharpening the perspective on how much time we have on this earth and how we are spending it. I've had to ask myself: Are you making sure you're not filling all your time just to fill all your time but treating time as a valuable resource and spending it well? Practically, that meant getting rid of activities that I did not enjoy or could be delegated or shortened and prioritizing activities that increased my joy and peace. I've learned not to take on so much that I have no time left for me or the people and things I truly care about. I reflect every day so I can pick up before I fall into problems.

PRACTICING WHAT I PREACH

As a manager, I've tried to accommodate my staff so that they always feel free to take their vacations and whatever time off is needed to care for their loved ones. I was always pro-work-life balance when it came to my staff, especially the parents. As a mother, I knew how important it was to put your kid on the bus in the morning. I would be the first to tell a nurse it's okay to come in later and just be flexible so that my staff could have that good balance of family and work.

When I first became a nurse manager for the ICU several years ago, it was two years-plus before I took vacation because, back then, I felt this sense of personal responsibility to make sure everything was running smoothly and didn't want to entrust my work to anyone else. I had set some milestones that needed to be reached before I could feel comfortable going away on vacation. Back when Blackberries were a thing, I would be the person constantly checking messages and answering them right away. It took many long years to learn I don't have to react to every message or every beep. We have to learn to set proper boundaries; otherwise, you could work yourself to the bone. Sometimes it's not that people are asking us to do it. We just put that extra pressure on ourselves.

PRIORITIZING MY PASSIONS

I have always traveled back to Jamaica at least once every year. Recently, I was able to travel back on a special trip. Northwell donated $820,000 of medical supplies and equipment to Jamaica in a partnership with medical nonprofit MedShare, and I was ecstatic to be part of that. I have also participated in community engagements educating Jamaicans about the COVID-19 vaccines and participating on panels at the University of the West Indies. I also attended my thirty-eighth high school reunion and was so pleased to see my old classmates.

My passion for health-care equity has meant that I spend many nights in hotels and hours on planes—which is time away from my precious grandson, my garden, and my treasured daily walks. But it is worth it. I love to know that I am making a difference. There are many problems in society that I cannot solve: racism, misogyny, sexism, socioeconomic disadvantages, ableism, and more. But in my specialty area of health care, I can do something, and I truly am happy to do it.

So, what works for you? Many women never get to a point of rest in their lives. Some die quite young of heart diseases, diabetes, hypertension, and certain cancers. Others live their lives managing these illnesses, unable to fully enjoy all the things they worked so hard for in their twenties, thirties, and forties. I will not burden you with more statistics, but speak to your friends and family members about their lives. Many of us want more free time, less stress, and better health. We want to lose weight and have better, more fulfilling relationships. Some might be like me and want more experiences and challenges. I might want to have a farm and raise chickens or start a foundation to benefit women and school-age children in New York City and across Jamaica. Sometimes we feel we have no control over these things, so we work because at least that is under our control. But is that really the case? Are we really doomed to lives of overwork and busyness, taking care of everyone else's needs while ours go unmet? Can we, especially as we hit middle age and older, put a stop to the madness?

WHAT WORKS FOR ME

Caring for myself means knowing what works for me and doing those things as often as possible so I can feel restored and fulfilled after a lifetime of hard work and self-sacrifice. Returning home frequently to Jamaica has always provided a refuge from the stress of America. As I have shared before, I enjoy beauty and fashion. Now that I travel more and attend more events on a national and international scale, I enjoy having my makeup and hair done and shopping for and wearing beautiful clothes. It's not for everybody, but a glamorous transformation certainly brings me a lot of joy when I go out on the town with friends or family. Even though I remain an introvert, I hardly ever turn down invitations to social events. I have found that they energize me, and when I get all dolled up, I feel confident and powerful.

Once I was able to buy my first home, I made sure there was enough room for a garden. Even though my grandparents had acres of green, fertile land, I grew up hating gardening. For one thing, watering the plants cut into my time to play. And I hated to get my hands dirty, girly girl that I was back then. However, I developed a love for gardening from my friend Pauline. I would visit her home and be awestruck by her beautiful garden and her knack for creative container gardening, year after year producing the most beautiful blooms. Pauline and I bonded over traveling far and wide to procure the most unusual plants.

Pre-COVID-19, when life was simpler and we had more time, my friend Pauline and I traveled to Litchfield, Connecticut, every year to buy unusual hostas, Japanese grass, and coral bells in colors we couldn't find locally. We would hunt down plants with great foliage, textures, and blooms for container gardening. Twombly Nursery never disappointed. It was like a girls' day trip for us. The car was filled to the brim, every inch in the trunk, back seat, the floor, and even in Pauline's lap. Pauline is a master at container gardening; it is an art, and I have learned so much from her.

I also fell in love with the idea of watching things grow from a seed, a dried piece of bark, or what looked like lifeless roots. It might sound cliché, but gardening, like walking, became an escape from the busyness and stress of life, a form of therapy. I always feel restored, calm, and joyful after spending time with my bare hands in the soil. The more I've gotten into gardening, the more possibilities it has opened up for me. I also love to eat what I grow; the best-tasting vegetables and greens I've tasted in America have come from my own soil.

I couldn't have pursued this hobby while living in a sixth-floor walk-up in the Bronx at nineteen years old. But many of you reading this do have the ability to decide today to add a restorative activity to your life so that you are being replenished and restored. Are you taking the time to do what it takes to work for yourself instead of others?

NEW YORK, NEW YORK

I'll always come back to New York, no matter where I go. I don't know if I could ever leave New York permanently, not even for my first love, Jamaica. I love the fast pace, the people, the cutting-edge fashion, busyness, everything about it. I also love the diversity. I have traveled quite extensively, and let me tell you, as a Black woman, I feel at home in New York more than any other state in the country. Of course, I know that racism exists in the city and beyond. But I have found that in its own unique, tough-love way, New York can offer people of color insulation from racism by its scrappy, individualistic ethic and respect for those who work hard. If you can make it here, you belong, no matter your background.

SEEING THE WORLD

One of the ways I have broadened my perspective of the world and even healed some of the racism I have experienced in America is by traveling. I have traveled to several countries with family and friends. And each time, it has been a learning experience and deeply fulfilling. Europe and Africa were among my top trips. I fell in love with Tanzania, Kenya, Ethiopia, and South Africa, which I visited for my fiftieth birthday. Each country was different and special in its own way. It was a pricey trip but so worth it to experience the different cultures of the African diaspora.

Garfield, as well, in his own words, would tell you that traveling as a Black man has been another way to embrace himself and to see himself outside the perspective of America and its complicated history. "I encourage young people to explore and go to places," Garfield says, adding that sometimes it costs less to go to a foreign country than to travel in the United States. Sometimes we can face prejudice and ignorance outside the US. Food research comes in handy. Know before you go. Ask people for their reviews. And just because one person or one influencer had a bad experience in one part of a single country doesn't mean that will be the same for everyone who goes there. Garfield intends to keep traveling and has visited all the continents except Antarctica. Needless to say, I'm ready to pack my bags and a puffy jacket. Let's go!

CHAPTER 33

On Our Own: Not the
Way It's Supposed to Be

You may have heard of the loneliness epidemic, as probably thousands of articles have been written about it in the last few years. Thirty or forty years ago, it probably would have seemed strange to connect a lack of social connection with physiological outcomes, but here we are. In 2023, the US surgeon general declared loneliness an epidemic, saying it poses a health risk as serious as stroke and heart disease. Not only that, but loneliness affects the young and the old, every ethnic group and social class.[71]

During COVID-19, I definitely felt the physical isolation from the lockdowns, and living alone only made it worse. I was busy with work and finishing up my doctorate. But I still felt disconnected and craved the natural human connections I had previously taken for granted—for

---

[71] "Surgeon General Declares Loneliness Epidemic, Saying It Poses Risks as Deadly as Smoking," CBS News, May 4, 2023, https://www.cbsnews.com/news/loneliness-surgeon-general-epidemic-covid/.

example, sitting at Starbucks on a Sunday morning and people-watching. My mother, my brother, my son, and other family members have always lived nearby, a short drive or a phone call away. Through difficult times, like my childbirth, my short marriage and subsequent divorce, and my career highs and lows, I have always been able to stop by Mom's to vent or have Garfield over for advice and counsel. During the pandemic, when we were all isolating, it was terribly painful how much I missed those connections. We could still talk on the phone, but I desperately missed eating together and being physically close to my mother especially.

For some, there is no loneliness epidemic because COVID-19 forced their families back together. Young professionals moved back home to remote work from their parents' and grandparents' homes. Roommates who hardly saw each other before the pandemic had to learn how to share space. Some kids who hardly ever saw their busy, working parents together were now sharing dinner as a family. But, according to health agencies, this constant togetherness is not the norm for too many of us, and loneliness can pose a serious risk.

"The physical health consequences of poor or insufficient connection include a 29% increased risk of heart disease, a 32% increased risk of stroke, and a 50% increased risk of developing dementia for older adults. Additionally, lacking social connection increases risk of premature death by more than 60%," according to the surgeon general's report.[72] A recent statement from the American Heart Association warned that social isolation and loneliness are linked to a 30 percent increased risk of heart attack, stroke, or death from either.[73] In the same statement, the AHA stated that the risk of social isolation increases with age due to life factors such as widowhood and retirement.

---

[72] "New Surgeon General Advisory Raises Alarm about the Devastating Impact of the Epidemic of Loneliness and Isolation in the United States," US Department of Health and Human Services, May 3, 2023, https://www.hhs.gov/about/news/2023/05/03/new-surgeon-general-advisory-raises-alarm-about-devastating-impact-epidemic-loneliness-isolation-united-states.html.

[73] "Social Isolation and Loneliness Increase the Risk of Death from Heart Attack, Stroke," American Heart Association, August 4, 2022, https://newsroom.heart.org/news/social-isolation-and-loneliness-increase-the-risk-of-death-from-heart-attack-stroke.

During COVID-19, many of the sickest patients and the ones who ultimately died were the elderly. Sometimes, they were brought into the hospital by family, but a lot of the time, they came from long-term care facilities. It was sad to witness the rates of death of the elderly across the country, knowing that many died isolated from loved ones. For the elderly who did survive the virus, going home from the hospital presented particular challenges. Even for younger patients who lived alone, discharging them posed problems. COVID-19 patients usually were sent home with a care protocol that required the help of a loved one, depending on how sick the patient had been, someone to take their temperature, measure their blood oxygen, and, if they had been on a ventilator, to provide overall monitoring. If the patient did not have someone to care for them, it often meant they had to remain hospitalized for a longer period.

I often thought of people who lived alone during the early weeks of the pandemic when emergency rooms and ambulance services were overwhelmed by the volume of infected. At one point in April 2020, the medical examiner's office in New York was reporting that two hundred city residents were dying at home each day, compared to twenty to twenty-five such deaths before the pandemic.[74] The New York metro has such a global population, and I wondered how people estranged from their families and with few close relationships outside of work were faring. The pandemic, in yet another unexpected way, exposed how the disconnectedness of our lives can endanger our health.

OUR BUSY, DISTRACTED CULTURE

Let's face it: our culture has not given a lot of support for family time, certainly not with demanding work schedules and increasing costs of living competing for even the most dedicated parents' time with their kids.

---

[74] Gwynne Hogan, "Staggering Surge of NYers Dying in Their Homes Suggests City Is Undercounting Coronavirus Fatalities," *Gothamist*, April 7, 2020, https://gothamist.com/news/surge-number-new-yorkers-dying-home-officials-suspect-undercount-covid-19-related-deaths.

There's no point in longing for the old days when families could thrive on just one parent's salary, leaving mom or dad home to care for the children and greet them after school with a hug and homemade snack. Those days are not coming back—if they ever existed. And I won't even get into how much social media has sapped our precious attention spans. We've traded away time with loved ones for the solace of a screen. Indeed, being physically at home does not necessarily equal emotional presence.

WE'RE NOT DOING GREAT

A friend of mine had a birthday recently, and to put it mildly, she was not excited. "Why aren't you excited about turning sixty-three?" I asked her. "You have so much to be grateful for."

But she didn't want to hear the Pollyanna pep talk. "I don't want to be ungrateful," she replied. "I'm just thinking about aging. I'm having aches and pains and health issues."

Aging is not fun, she added, especially when you're single and crave companionship.

I felt her pain, and I understand the impulse to burrow into our funky moods and shut out the world when these thoughts fight for space in our minds. I'm of the mindset that we should feel all of our feelings. We should know by now that ignoring and burying those emotions does not benefit our minds, bodies, or souls.

But how long should we wallow, especially if the problem is something we can act on, even in some small way? "That's not the way to live," I told my friend. I encouraged her to take the time to feel all her feelings but to not linger too long in the pit! I asked her questions: What can we do about the pain? Are you getting enough sleep and exercise? Did you call your doctor? That's what I would want from a friend when I'm down in the dumps. Pick me up. Talk me out of it!

Life is not going to be perfect, even if you're young, fit, rich, and beautiful. Something is always wrong because this world is not heaven! But there is always hope, and when we look around, there is plenty to be grateful for. Sometimes, all we need to do is get up and go outside and figuratively and literally get outside of ourselves.

I encourage anyone who is tempted to withdraw inward to try to get out and be social. You may not make any friends, but you will have experiences. Some might be hilarious, some life-changing, and some you might want to forget. But I believe all of that is part of living. It doesn't have to be a garden or other type of club. It can be a volunteer opportunity to work with young people or help seniors or serve your community. There are plenty of opportunities out there that can take us outside of the house and train our focus on something beyond ourselves.

DEATHS OF DESPAIR

For several years, the rising rate of people dying from alcohol-related liver diseases, drug overdoses, and suicides, particularly the effects of the opioid addiction crisis, has included largely White Americans.[75] However, in recent years, new research has shown that people of color, including Native Americans, are also at risk for these "deaths of despair."

A recent report from the CDC[76] marked an increase in 2021 suicide rates nationally after two consecutive years of declines. That report had some startling news for communities of color. During 2018–2021, age-adjusted suicide rates increased significantly for Black people from 7.3 to 8.7, a 19.2 percent increase, and for Hispanic persons from 7.4 to 7.9, a 6.8 percent increase. The only group to show an overall age-adjusted rate decline compared with that in 2018 (from 18.1 to 17.4, a 3.9 percent decline) was White Americans. The report also showed a sharp increase in the rate of suicide for young Black people aged 10–24 years from 8.2 to 11.2; a 36.6 percent increase).

[75] Rhitu Chatterjee, "Native Americans Left Out of 'Deaths of Despair' Research," NPR, February 1, 2023, https://www.npr.org/sections/health-shots/2023/02/01/1152222968/native-americans-left-out-of-deaths-of-despair-research.

[76] Deborah M. Stone et al., "Notes from the Field: Recent Changes in Suicide Rates, by Race and Ethnicity and Age Group — United States, 2021," *Morbidity and Mortality Weekly Report*, 72, no. 6 (February 10, 2023): 160–62, https://www.cdc.gov/mmwr/volumes/72/wr/mm7206a4.htm.

The pandemic was a tipping point for people who were living on the edge financially, emotionally, mentally, and in so many other ways. The social, economic, and relational impact of the COVID-19 years took what little hope and stability was left for people already struggling with loneliness or other hardships. The economy may seem strong and the unemployment rate low, but many people lost jobs and coworker relationships during the pandemic. Even more lost small businesses that they'd worked very hard to build. With a million Americans lost to the virus, we continue to have a nation of mourners.

The fact is, there was reason to despair before and particularly after the pandemic. Sometimes when I see videos online of people acting out in public, I wonder what brought them to that point of anger, to losing their natural restraint. Other people may not act out in public, but the numbers of suicides and drug and alcohol addiction tell the story. The question now is: How do we come back from the pandemic and recover from our emotional and health losses? Is there a role for the government to play? Is there a role for the health-care industry, for communities, and for families to play? Yes, to all of the above!

It is encouraging to see the loss of the stigma associated with seeking mental help, especially in the Black community. For too long, we have stigmatized mental illness and not taken advantage of the help available to us. Young or old, we must realize that seeking mental health care is as basic as taking Tylenol for a headache. There should be no shame in it.

SAFEGUARDING OUR CONNECTIONS

As a busy professional and single mother, loneliness has never been a huge issue for me, except during COVID-19, as I've shared. The pandemic exacerbated a lot of our social, economic, and political problems, and the aftermath of COVID-19 is also contributing to the social and psychological hardship felt by many. It is nothing to be ashamed of, and we should feel empowered to speak about our loneliness and the healing benefits of social connection with as much passion as we do about eating right and exercising. Those of us who have families and social connections would do well to guard those connections and nurture them, as much as we would see eating well and exercise as ways to maintain our health.

Like me, you might want to blame social media, smartphones, and a faster pace of life for our disconnected, lonely lives. But those are not the only culprits. We must intentionally choose relationships, sometimes even at the cost of our career or financial advancement. To choose to be with family even when it's not perfect, even when we may have to give a bit more of ourselves than we want to, is worth it. These interactions help us train our patience and grace muscles! Plus, if we keep in mind our own imperfections, it's easier to be patient with others' imperfections. Relationships are difficult, but in most cases, they are worth our time and could benefit our health in the long run.

COMMUNITY IS HEALTHY

As a young woman working hard to pay bills and become acclimated to American culture, I desperately missed the close-knit community I grew up in. To me, America offered unlimited opportunities for economic mobility, but there was a cost. As I scarfed down quick, unhealthy meals, I longed for the slow, healthy dinners of my childhood and the conversations with my grandparents and other family during those meals.

My new life meant I was too busy for those types of meals; for one thing, I worked on Sundays. I can see how easy it is to be trapped in the cycle of hard work and achievement while social connections slowly fade away.

But you don't need a big family—or a dining table, for that matter. Good health means connecting with other humans, whether in our churches or other faith communities, community and neighborhood groups, volunteer organizations, or through hobbies. The ways in which we connected in the past seem to be going out of fashion. But, please, let's bring that back! A US Health and Human Services Report showed that since the 1970s, religious preference, affiliation, and participation among US adults declined. "In 2020, only 47% of Americans said they belonged to a church, synagogue, or mosque. This is down from 70% in 1999 and represents a dip below 50% for the first time in the history of the survey question."[77] The HHS report notes that a sense of belonging around shared values and beliefs is associated with reduced risk-taking behaviors, which can lead to poorer health outcomes. I don't go to church every single Sunday, but I do make it a point to attend and be a part of a faith community. It's one of the free, easy, and rewarding ways to know and be known by a community of like-minded people. In some communities, churches and other faith centers are literally on every other corner. There has to be one that works for you.

THE VALUE OF COMMUNITY: A CASE STUDY

My grandmother, as I mentioned earlier, suffered from diabetes and hypertension for decades. I was very involved in her care as an adolescent, along with my siblings. Caring for her solidified for me that I wanted to be a nurse. My grandmother was an inspiration for the many students she taught and in the Anglican church, where she served as organist and director of the Sunday school. Her home was also the meeting spot for our community youth club, so our house was always full of people. Because of my father, people from our community were always coming to our house for one reason or another. You would think that my grandmother came from a large family or had a large family herself, but that was not the case. There was just my father and his older brother, who lived in England. My grandparents' wealth of connections came from the community, which they lived and breathed and invested in for their entire lives.

In addition to our family connections, we attended church several times a week, forming a familial bond with our church community.

---

[77] "Our Epidemic of Loneliness and Isolation: The U.S. Surgeon General's Advisory on the Healing Effects of Social Connection and Community," US Department of Health and Human Services, 2023, https://www.hhs.gov/sites/default/files/surgeon-general-social-connection-advisory.pdf.

There were also youth sports and civic clubs in our May Pen community that my siblings and I joined.

I am trying to paint a picture of community, family, and connectedness, which I think has always been very important for our communities in the diaspora, whether in the brick buildings of the Bronx, suburban backyards in Maryland, or small towns in the Mississippi Delta. We should treasure those family and community bonds because they are medicine for our souls. I am not saying we should maintain toxic family relationships, mind you. I am saying there is treasure in relationships and a sense of community, and if we are blessed to have them, we should not throw them away.

CARING FOR MY GRANDMOTHER AS A FAMILY

I believe my grandmother lived long, even with her disease, because she was surrounded by family who participated in her care, and she was able to live in her home and community around the people and things she loved and valued.

More people are diagnosed and are living long, productive lives with diabetes, but many are also dying or suffering from complications, such as amputations. My family was fortunate in that we could all work together on my grandmother's behalf, down to how the food was prepared. Everyone in our household was sympathetic to her not being able to eat certain things, and I believe that inspired us kids to eat healthier as well. My grandmother was able to live with her chronic illness while teaching, playing the organ in church, and leading in all of her community activities. I believe the family support had a lot to do with the rich and full life she lived.

CHOOSING THE HEALTHIEST PHYSICAL— AND EMOTIONAL—ADDRESS

I get it, trust me! Some members of our families are full of drama and negativity. And that's where we learn to draw boundary lines, reclaim, protect, and preserve our peace! But it shouldn't be so easy and natural for us to cut off our familial and communal bonds with the people who have known us the longest and probably the best.

Some people who moved across the country for jobs or school found themselves terrified during the pandemic of what would happen to them or distant family in case of infection and serious sickness. Now may be a good time to inventory our lives to determine whether the choices we have made in where we live and who we live close to make sense for our health.

That suburban community, while beautiful, came with drawbacks. The houses were spaced far enough apart that I never got to know my neighbors, and people tended to keep to themselves. My neighbors were mostly cordial and welcoming, but it was hard to connect. Their kids were much younger than Kadeem, for instance. So, on the street, he didn't have any friends. There just wasn't the sense of community I needed.

Since then, I've been very thoughtful about where I live and where I put down my roots. I've lived in tiny apartments and big houses. None of that matters to me anymore. Quality of life matters to me. And my experiences in life as I grow older matter to me.

It's not just about a house with the square footage, picket fence, or curb appeal. What goes into my list of considerations are: Is it diverse? Is it walkable? Is it safe? How is the town governed? Is there a sense of community? Does a community have a voice? Who are the leaders locally and on the state and federal level? All those things matter to me, especially during this time of political polarization. I certainly wouldn't just up and move to another state simply because of lower home prices. There's so much more going into that equation. So, I continue to choose New York—it checks all my boxes.

START WITH ONE PERSON

During the height of the COVID-19 crisis, as close as I am to my family, it was my work colleague who I made a pact with for my care if I ever got the virus. My good friend Debra is a single woman, an Irish American nurse who worked with me for years before moving on to another institution. We were both working hard during COVID-19 and shared our fears of getting infected. We decided that if either of us became seriously sick, we would care for each other because we were both single and about age fifty. The plan was she would move into her basement, and I would live upstairs in her house to care for her while she was sick. If I got sick, then she would do the same for me. It seems comical and dramatic now that that pandemic is over. But we were a fantastic mutual support system in 2020. We spent a lot of time together, taking long walks, playing with her dog Maggie, and cooking elaborate dinners, pretending we were dining at fancy restaurants.

Once the crisis abated, she made positive changes in her life that were not that great for me. For one, she returned home to Ireland to be closer to her aging parents. I miss her being close by, but I understand her desire to be home with her family. It is a natural feeling.

It is worth considering whether where you are is the best place to age, to live as a single person, or as a young family desperately in need of help from your parents and siblings. All these are questions that can determine your health and quality of life.

A SADDER OUTCOME

Social isolation can have dire consequences. One family friend, who I'll call John, also an immigrant from the West Indies, was diagnosed with diabetes in his thirties. This was a vibrant young man who loved reggae music, watching soccer games, and cooking and who was a dedicated employee. He had been single his entire life but saw his extended family regularly toward the end of his life. The first few years in America for working-class immigrants can be brutal as we seek to achieve the goals that brought us to the land of opportunity. It was no different for John, who lived in the same home with his extended family during his first decade in the US. Through his jobs, John was able to get good health insurance and access to great doctors. He was put on insulin in his mid-thirties, and his doctors encouraged him to eat healthier and exercise, which he did for the next several years.

However, as the years went by, his health began to slip again. He had experienced a painful breakup with a woman, and the closeness in the extended family began to fray when he moved to his own place. He no longer had his older sisters to check on him daily, to ask him if he was taking his medications, and to make sure he was eating the right foods. He was still very connected to his coworkers, however. As a matter of fact, it was a nurse at his job who encouraged him to take his medications and even helped him figure out the apparatus for administering insulin to himself.

When COVID-19 hit in March 2020, his life changed within days. His connections were lost as his job shut down. Because of the warnings to isolate, he stayed inside, not seeing family or friends. Unwisely, he stopped his medications. Unfortunately, and maybe unbeknownst to him, he was becoming dangerously ill. In early April 2020, he walked a few blocks in his neighborhood to visit a friend. He did not make it back to his apartment. He passed away from cardiac arrest related to diabetes. He did not have COVID-19, his autopsy showed. He was only fifty-nine.

Those of us who knew him were shocked. Some of us felt guilt. Why didn't we make sure he was taking his meds? What could we have done differently? We are still mourning our friend. And we are aware enough to make sure we do a better job of checking in and sending a text to say, "What's up? How are you today?"

I think back to Dr. Arline Geronimus's work on "weathering" when I compare my grandmother's long life in Jamaica, even with hypertension and diabetes, and the relatively short life of John and other immigrants in the US who experience the same chronic diseases and shorter life expectancies of our American-born Black brothers and sisters. None of us are immune from the psychobiological burdens of living as a person of color in America. We must be vigilant to look out for ourselves and each other; our lives depend on it.

BUILD A MORE CONNECTED LIFE

The challenges in our society today are so overwhelming that I can't even begin to think of a solution, but I like what the surgeon general advises. We already have the community infrastructure—churches, libraries, and community centers—that we can strengthen to foster those connections with our neighbors. Volunteering with seniors, mentoring youth, or getting involved with a place of worship, faith organizations, and sporting and exercise groups are just some ways we can remain connected to others in our community and work toward ending the loneliness epidemic.

Part V

THE POWER
OF POSSIBILITY

CHAPTER 34

Passing It Down, Paying It Forward

T he Girl Scouts of Suffolk County are a fun bunch of people! These young women recently had me drawing on the streets with chalk and playing double Dutch. It was the most fun I've had in a long time. I had delivered the keynote address at their Making an Impact breakfast event, so I was familiar with the leadership there. But at this particular summer event, they were honoring me in a way I still can't fully appreciate. They were celebrating "Sandra Lindsay Day."

The Nassau and Suffolk County executives Bruce Blakeman and Steve Bellone held a ceremony in Suffolk County on July 18, 2022, declaring it Sandra Lindsay Day in both counties in perpetuity. To commemorate the first anniversary of SLD, I decided to spend July 18, 2023, with the Girl Scouts. I enjoyed the carefree, joyous feelings these young ladies shared with me as we laughed and played together.

Investing in young people is one of the most fun parts of my work as a health-care advocate. Whether speaking to kids in Jamaica or New York City high schools, I am always energized and challenged by the younger generation. I've found their opinions to have weight and value that constantly challenge my worldview. Age and experience give us wisdom our youth have yet to acquire, but we can still learn a lot from them.

I try to never turn down an opportunity to speak at graduations, especially at community colleges and high schools. Who would have thought I would be on stage at Hofstra delivering a commencement speech and getting an honorary doctorate? This former struggling student, who was so shy and lacking in confidence, would have never imagined such a future for herself. Now that I have found my voice, I want other young girls and women to know they can overcome those awkward years—hopefully sooner than I did.

ALL OUR KIDS

At a recent high school graduation party in Florida, surrounded by family and friends of a teen who was crossing the stage, a sense of gratitude overwhelmed me. Garfield and I were helping out in the kitchen of our friends' house, chopping the onions and preparing ingredients for the meal we were helping to prepare for Taylor Rose's party. I looked around, and everyone we loved was there: her mom, Marie; her father, Philip; her grandfather, Paul; and her sweet great-grandmother, Aunt Nellie, who are like family to me. Despite the decades between us, Taylor and I bonded over fashion on a recent friends and family cruise through Northern Europe. We would frequently show up to dinners dressed alike without planning the outfits. We had forged a connection, and I couldn't miss her big day for the world.

The fact is, I was exhausted during the graduation festivities! I was dead tired from work and other travel. But this young lady had personally asked me to attend her graduation. I made the effort because she was worth it to me, and I did not regret it one bit.

The deep sense of love and gratitude came from reflecting on my past. This young woman's college journey and graduation was a far cry from those lonely, grinding days of the late 1980s when I was trying so hard to make it in New York. I had finally come full circle, in a way, celebrating with her family her achievement and the fact that we, the older generation, were in a position to provide our kids the opportunities we didn't have. This was an intergenerational graduation ceremony; all our collective hard work had paid off. This is my wish for all of us: that we transfer a legacy of holistic good health to the younger generation so that they, too, can pass it on.

During the party, Taylor's mom, Marie, gave a tearful speech that brought me to tears, too. She thanked everyone for their overwhelming support, not just for attending Taylor's graduation but for encouraging and supporting her throughout the journey. Busy work schedules and travel meant that the parents were not always there when Taylor got home from school or to oversee homework, among other things, but the extended family of cousins, aunts, uncles, and close friends filled the gap. This amazing army of people was her village, a strong community of support that was rooting for her and pushing her on to the next level of life.

My son is in his mid-thirties with his own family now, so he doesn't need my mothering as much as he did in the past. But Taylor is among dozens of young women who reach out to me, wanting career advice or just wanting to have lunch to talk about life. What a privilege to get to share my experiences with these young people and hopefully make a positive impact on their lives.

Plugging into activities and organizations that expose us to young people can do wonders for our outlook and our health. Girl Scouts and Big Brothers Big Sisters are the well-known ones. But what about your local church youth group? Or a young mom in your neighborhood who might need your wisdom on raising her toddlers or getting her baby to sleep? It can be a mutually rewarding alliance. Yes, they will help you figure out your new cell phone, but most likely, you both will gain something more relationally valuable.

THE NEXT GENERATION OF NURSES

During COVID-19, I had the great fortune of working with some of the bravest, most dedicated young nurses. Some of these young women were recent graduates in their first-ever real-world job when the pandemic hit. What a way to begin a career in nursing! As I have shared, my beginnings as a nurse were not easy, but I don't know what I would have done if my career had begun in the middle of a global pandemic. I don't know that my resilience would have brought me this far.

I was impressed by their perseverance and their commitment to the patients. I am sure that many are still dealing with the emotional and mental effects of having to face the volume of very sick patients and the deaths of 2020–21. It would have been understandable if these young women had walked away from the hospital and from nursing altogether. Even veteran nurses like me were shaken by what we were seeing in the ICU every day. But these young women, for the most part, stayed and worked and dedicated themselves to caring for our patients.

When I visit the floors and see these young nurses growing in their careers, I have nothing but the utmost admiration for them. These young men and women will be terrific leaders if they stay the course. We faced many challenges together, cried a lot, shared our disappointments, and celebrated minor victories like seeing a patient get off a ventilator or being discharged from the ICU.

Nursing is a challenging profession, I tell young people, but it can be immensely rewarding. At the bedside, you must get up close and personal with another human being: touching, cleaning, bathing them, administering medicine, turning them over in bed, and befriending them and their loved ones. Nursing requires a special type of person; you literally must be willing to get your hands dirty. But the rewards are there, and these young nurses are part of that reward for me. They are not quitters. They are vulnerable, professional, brilliant, funny, and excellent caregivers. My hope is to see them raise up another generation of young nurses in that same spirit of excellence.

CHAPTER 35

The Power of Possibility: From Grassroots to the Top

I n January 2023, I, along with OB/GYN physicians, an anesthesiol-ogist medical student, and my brother Garfield, a respiratory thera-pist, embarked on a surgical mission trip to Jamaica. The aim was to help clear a backlog of surgeries in Jamaica at the request of the minister of health. We brought loads of equipment along with our experience and expertise. It was not easy. We faced a mountain of paperwork navigating the licensing requirements, the differences in the health-care system, and the fact that many of us had not worked together before. But we were united by our belief and commitment to what we were doing. To be able to bring our American resources to these underserved hospitals and patients was a major win, not just for the patients but for us as well. I had always wanted an opportunity to give back to Jamaica, and this trip was, in a way, coming full circle for me. I know the rest of the team felt as proud of the work we did on that surgical mission trip.

Looking back on my experience with dengue fever as a twelve-year-old and my brother's battle with stomach cancer while living in Jamaica,

I see how health disparities can play out on a global scale. The health-care system in Jamaica is more modern and developed than in some other developing countries, but it still has a long way to go. I have been privileged to use my position to contribute to hospitals, schools, and in other ways—something I hope to do more of in the future.

What has been immensely satisfying to me is to see health-care professionals, communities, students, and people from all walks of life become energized in the fight for equitable health care for all. Each of us can play a role, no matter how minor, in addressing health-care disparities, whether by starting a community garden that grows fresh vegetables, mentoring a teenager, spending time with the elderly in a nursing home, or giving to great organizations that promote good health.

POLITICAL ROADBLOCKS

I hate politics. Because of my family's experience with political violence in Jamaica, I have always stayed far away from Jamaican politics, even though those tumultuous days are ancient history. The Jamaican political system and culture are certainly not perfect, but we have come a long way from the unrest of the 1980s and early 1990s. Even so, I carry my scars quite consciously. I tense up when people connect my name with my father's or when they assume that it's because of my last name that I became the first person to take the COVID-19 vaccine. The conspiracy theories can run deep and silly. Some people have even said that I received a big payoff for taking the vaccine. Trust me, I did not.

When I arrived in America in 1986, the fear of politics didn't leave me. Every election back home, I would be terrified, unable to sleep, worried for my family down there. American politics seemed like a Sunday picnic compared to what I had seen in Jamaica. In 1986, Ronald Reagan was president, and although I heard grumblings about him around my Bronx neighborhood, no one was threatening violence to their neighbors because of who they voted for. In the 1988, 1992, and 1996 elections, it was the same orderly, democratic process. I thought, "Wow! People can just cast their votes, and there's no shooting, killing, or fighting?

You don't have to be worried about what color you're wearing because it might offend the other party? I'll take that every day!"

Of course, the last few years in America have left a lot of us doubtful and a little afraid. Will we fall further into division and violence, or can we go back to those days of agreeing to disagree? I don't have the answers. What I saw on the news on that gray day in January 2021 sent shivers down my spine. The angry, violent protesters at the US Capitol were terrifying, and they stirred up memories of those horrible years of political violence in Jamaica.

"This is not the United States that I know, that I came to!" I lamented with a colleague at work. He is Haitian Dominican but has lived on Long Island since he was a child. He shook his head. "That's always been there," he said of the violence. He recounted the violence he and his family encountered in the early 1980s and the 1970s as one of the few people of color in his Long Island neighborhood. "For some reason," he said, "people are just emboldened now to act out what's always been in their hearts."

Could this be true? I wondered. But it seemed the events of 2020, the pandemic, the social unrest, and the election had combined to bring out the worst in so many of us. In my thirty-plus years in America, I had never seen the political atmosphere so polarized. For many who survived worse during the civil rights era and before, it must have felt like déjà vu.

In any democracy, there is a place for disagreement and righteous anger. That's just part of politics. What shouldn't be part of political debates are public goods that benefit us all, like equitable health care, particularly for those who need it the most. For instance, states should not be preventing federal health-care funding from reaching their poorest citizens because of ideological differences with who is or was in the White House. And presidential candidates should not be building their campaigns on rancor around vaccine or mask mandates. We have more pressing health problems in our communities that, if addressed, can ensure a healthier generation of voting Americans in the future.

WE NEED SOLUTIONS

It was discouraging in the summer of 2023 to see COVID-19 cases begin to surge as hot temperatures drove many people inside to air-conditioned buildings. Not again, I thought. But there were worse headlines of the summer: The US suicide rate had climbed 2.6 percent from 2021 to 2022, according to the CDC. The suicide rate for women had increased by 3.8 percent and was up 3.6 percent for Blacks/African Americans. Thankfully, the rate among youths had decreased by a healthy 8.4 percent, and the rate was down 6 percent for Native Americans.[78] But clearly, three years after the pandemic, we, as a nation, were still not doing okay.

As of the summer of 2023, some cities were still experiencing high crime rates, and high interest rates were causing fears of a recession. The end of the COVID-19 emergency meant that millions of people have been rolled off Medicaid[79] and other programs that provided health, food, and housing assistance. In 2023, experts saw a record increase in homeless people, up roughly 11 percent from 2022 and the biggest recorded increase since the government started tracking such numbers in 2007.[80] It's during times like these, when disheartening news headlines are pervasive, that our communities can begin to lose hope that the help that is desperately needed by the most vulnerable will soon disappear for good.

DOING THE WORK OURSELVES

Unfortunately, it seems that a lot of the policy solutions we need to address many of the problems we face in our community are intertwined with politics—so much so that it can be difficult to get things done. But

---

[78] "Suicide Data and Statistics," Centers for Disease Control and Prevention, https://www.cdc.gov/suicide/suicide-data-statistics.html.

[79] "Medicaid Enrollment and Unwinding Tracker," KFF, August 14, 2023, https://www.kff.org/medicaid/issue-brief/medicaid-enrollment-and-unwinding-tracker/.

[80] Jon Kamp and Shannon Najmabadi, "More Americans Are Ending Up Homeless—at a Record Rate," *Wall Street Journal*, August 14, 2023, https://www.wsj.com/articles/homelessness-increasing-united-states-housing-costs-e1990ac7.

I believe some things are changing for the better. I see examples of it daily in my work at Northwell and as I talk to people from all walks of life about what they are doing to make our society more equitable.

The problems facing our communities go from the womb to the tomb. I have discussed the startling infant mortality rate for Black babies in America. Experts have noted that children who grow up in substandard inner-city housing have worse health outcomes, such as complications from asthma, compared to children in more affluent areas where health-care access is greater or of higher quality. We could say the same for food insecurity, lack of proper access to grocery stores, and the like. For instance, the area in the Bronx, where I lived when I first emigrated, had a lot of fast food establishments, and small grocery stores that did not carry a wide array of fresh fruits of vegetables. Many of our communities are not safe enough for people to walk around or for kids to play in the park. These issues all contribute to poor health indicators. We need a national conversation on how to address these issues and improve the health of those in our nation at the bottom of the socioeconomic ladder.

When I think of policy solutions, I think of what I would have liked to have seen in my lower-income Bronx neighborhood back in the '80s and '90s. Recently, when I had the opportunity to speak with Tony Hillery, founder and CEO of Harlem Grown, I thought, "There's something a community can do without much help from public officials and/or toxic politics!" Hillery founded his nonprofit Harlem Grown in 2011 to address the health and academic challenges facing public elementary school students in Harlem. He started his urban farming initiative in an abandoned lot across from elementary school P.S. 175. Now, 13 years later Harlem Grown has matured into a network of thirteen urban farms ranging from soil-based farms, hydroponic greenhouses, and school gardens that harvest thousands of pounds of fresh produce a year. And that number is growing and growing. I can mentally check off all the problems that this initiative potentially targets: food insecurity, environmental health, healthy eating, education, and keeping kids engaged and involved in their community. What a win for everyone.

GREENS AND COMMUNITY

I am so excited about this initiative that I have volunteered with Harlem Grown on several summer Saturdays at their farm stand. It was so rewarding! I simply signed up, got up, and took the train to 134th Street in Harlem.

The volunteer team put out tables for the produce, and I got busy with them. We tied up bunches of basil, Swiss chard, lettuce, and more. Then, there were piles of mushrooms, peppers, beets, tomatoes, and carrots. The mushrooms came in different varieties, including oyster and lion's mane. Don't forget, this was all grown by children, volunteers, and Harlem Grown staff in in an urban environment!

Oh, and it was free. All free. We just stood on the street corner, and as people walked up, they could get a bag of fresh food to take home. I was beside myself with joy to be a part of this. The people who volunteer and work there could also get a bag to take home. One woman came with a huge black garbage bag. "I have eight kids," she said. "This is so good." She was grateful to be able to take home these blessings for her family. Another great thing: there was no shame in any of this. Instead, there was a sense of joy and community. Folks rolled up on foot, nicely dressed, on Citi Bikes, men, women, young and old. It was wonderful. Some were regulars and were asking for their favorites. "Where is the arugula?" someone asked. Others asked, "Where's the corn?" Some were just passing by and stopped out of curiosity. Many couldn't believe this was all free.

The volunteers were dedicated and enthusiastic. The high school kids sometimes participate in the farm stand, but sometimes, college students and the community volunteer as well. That day, we had a successful farm stand, and over a hundred people showed up. Harlem Grown doesn't only grow stuff; it measures its success. There is a counter at the farm stand to keep track of the number of people benefiting from their work.

Even better is the education that takes place alongside all of this. There is a misperception that people in low-income areas are not interested in vegetables or in cooking healthy. But part of Harlem Grown's work has been educating the kids who grow the food on how to prepare it at home. "So, the kids now say, 'I like this type of mushroom and not this other type.'" They love arugula which is odd because it's kind of spicy, but Hillery said it is one of their favorite vegetables.

Tony Hillery's vision and persistence drive so much of these fantastic results. Tony will tell you that when Harlem Grown started, the kids and their parents couldn't identify some of the greens and vegetables. What Harlem Grown did was to host cooking classes at one of the gardens. Parents and kids came in and were shown how to prepare these foods. "If you educate people and make it available, they'll eat it," Tony has said. Isn't that amazing? Don't you want to see this all over America? I certainly do!

My dream is to see more of these programs in our cities and other areas affected by food insecurity. Harlem Grown began by surveying the area and knowing the community and its challenges. Tony Hillery didn't go to war with or try to get rid of fast-food restaurants. He simply gave the community a choice by incorporating fruits and vegetables into what was available to them. Healthy food was as prominent in their sightlines as fast food. Once the education part of it was done and the barrier of the unknown was overcome, folks could make better choices on what to eat. And now, that community lines up on summer Saturdays at 11 a.m. for healthy food.

Urban farming is just one of the many ways we can take a holistic approach to improve our personal health and the health of our communities. Holistic approaches to health-care equity take more than increasing the number of grocery stores or adding bike lanes and parks in our neighborhoods. It also means safe and secure housing free of lead and other toxins, clean drinking water, better access to public transportation, and community leaders who listen, interact, and act with members of the community.

MATERNAL AND INFANT CARE

The distressing statistics on black infant mortality and the health risks Black women face during and after childbirth highlight the dangers of childbearing in America. Thanks to the work of journalists like Linda Villarosa, those awful statistics are not going unnoticed, and a few cities and states have begun taking action to address inequities in maternal and postpartum care. For instance, as of mid-2022, six states (Oregon, Minnesota, New Jersey, Florida, Maryland, and Virginia) reimbursed Medicaid patients for doula services, just one area that could help women have safe and healthy deliveries. As we know, the problem is much bigger and needs a holistic solution focused on promoting life and ensuring that disadvantaged children and families thrive.

Corporations and nonprofits are also getting in on the act. In Our Own Voice: National Black Women's Reproductive Justice Agenda[81] is a national-state partnership focused on amplifying the voices of Black women leaders in the fight for reproductive justice. The organization has partnered with like-minded groups, including the Interfaith Voices for Reproductive Justice and SisterLove, Inc., in creating and releasing the Black Reproductive Justice Policy Agenda, created in collaboration with more than thirty Black women's organizations and reproductive justice activists. According to In Our Own Voice, the agenda discusses policy solutions and endorses key legislation about:

- Health equity, care, and access, including maternal health and pregnancy care, chronic health conditions, and behavioral and mental health.
- Social justice, community justice, and safety, including voting rights, police violence, gender-based violence, economic justice, education justice, LGBTQIA+ liberation, environmental justice, and housing justice.

---

[81] "Black Reproductive Policy Agenda," Our Own Voice: National Black Women's Reproductive Justice Agenda, https://blackrj.org/blackrjpolicy/.

- Religion and reproductive justice and the role faith and spirituality have played in countering efforts to control Black women, girls, and gender-expansive people's sexuality and bodily autonomy.

In the US Congress, positive change has been brought about by the Black Maternal Health Caucus led by Congresswomen Alma Adams of North Carolina and Lauren Underwood of Illinois. The US House of Representatives approved in the fiscal year 2022 omnibus appropriations package multiple priorities of the Black Maternal Health Caucus,[82] including:

- $83 million for Safe Motherhood/Infant Health Programs at the Centers for Disease Control and Prevention, which include Maternal Mortality Review Committees and Perinatal Quality Collaboratives.
- $30 million for the National Institute of Health Implementing a Maternal Health and Pregnancy Outcomes Vision for Everyone (IMPROVE), an unprecedented investment in the flagship maternal health research initiative at NIH.
- $748 million, an increase of $35 million, for the Maternal and Child Health Block Grant to fund programs that support the health and well-being of mothers, children, and families. This flexible funding stream allows states to meet local maternal and child health needs, providing services to an estimated sixty million Americans every year.

The package also includes funding for maternal mental health programs, screening and treatment for maternal depression and related disorders, and appropriations targeted at maternal care in rural areas of the country.

---

[82] "Black Maternal Health Caucus Celebrates Inclusion of Nearly $1 Billion in Maternal Health Priorities in Appropriations Bill," Black Maternal Health Caucus, US House of Representatives, March 9, 2022, https://blackmaternalhealthcaucus-underwood.house.gov/media/press-releases/black-maternal-health-caucus-celebrates-inclusion-nearly-1-billion-maternal.

In May, Senator Cory Booker joined the effort to reintroduce the bicameral Black Maternal Health Momnibus Act.[83] "The United States has the highest maternal mortality rate of industrialized nations, and the rate is only rising. The data is even more concerning for Black moms," said Senator Booker. "No one deserves to be left behind by the health care system or face inadequate care during pregnancy, labor, and postpartum. This legislation is a critical step towards saving lives, ending disparities in health care and outcomes, and ensuring our health care system treats all moms with the care and dignity they deserve regardless of their race or circumstance. I am proud to join my colleagues in introducing this bill that would address the drivers of the maternal health crisis, invest in social determinants of health, and ensure comprehensive support for all people. It's time to prioritize the well-being of all, eliminate racial and ethnic disparities for Black and Brown moms, and create a brighter and healthier future for all families."

VACCINES, LEADING, AND EDUCATION

A couple of years ago, I taped a segment for the Department of Health and Human Services with Dr. Kizzmekia Corbett, a viral immunologist and one of the leading pioneers of the COVID-19 vaccines. Dr. Corbett continues to work on vaccine development for pandemic preparedness and is an assistant professor at the Harvard School of Public Health. One of the things we talked about was the importance of representation. Dr. Corbett noted that being a public face of the COVID-19 vaccines achieved just what it should have: it showed underrepresented communities that people who looked like them were involved in the research process for vaccines. In other words, her public-facing work had built trust. We talked about the fact that, unwittingly, we both had become

---

[83] "Booker, Underwood, Adams Reintroduce the Bicameral Momnibus Act to End America's Maternal Health Crisis," Cory Booker, May 15, 2023, https://www.booker.senate.gov/news/press/booker-underwood-adams-reintroduce-the-bicameral-momnibus-act-to-end-americas-maternal-health-crisis.

the inspiration for girls and women who now wanted to pursue careers in research, medicine, and nursing. Representation matters!

Dr. Corbett's work on coronavirus vaccines began way before the pandemic struck. In 2015, she and other scientists had begun creating experimental vaccines against SARS and MERS.[84] Dr. Corbett is among several rising scientists of color who are doing the work on vaccine preparedness and spreading the word in our communities. Their work will go a long way to prepare us for the next pandemic and to reverse our communities' centuries of mistrust in medicine.

FACING THE NEXT PANDEMIC

My hope is that we never have to face another pandemic, but that is an unrealistic hope, according to experts. So what can we do besides continue to develop vaccines and educate our communities? Well, the list is very long. Based on my COVID-19 experience, I would like to see a few things.

My CEO at Northwell outlined about a dozen priorities and steps to prepare for future vital steps that I would like to echo. Among them are issues near and dear to my heart—for example, building an emergency management culture in our government and institutions, urgently addressing inequities in health-care access, protecting the physical and emotional health of frontline workers, and reversing America's cultural disrespect for science.

If more health-care institutions invested in training and preparing their staff for events such as what we experienced in 2020–21, their staff might be better prepared for the toll a pandemic can take professionally and personally. Addressing the needs of nurses, doctors, administrators, and others could reverse the staffing shortages and burnout. The mental, professional, and physical health of frontline workers should be top priorities for our institutions.

---

[84] Debra Kamin, "She Helped Unlock the Science of the Covid Vaccine," *New York Times*, February 9, 2023, https://www.nytimes.com/2023/02/09/science/covid-vaccine-kizzmekia-corbett.html.

Educating the public is an ongoing mission that I am proud to be a part of in day-to-day work. Whether through hosting a podcast, public speaking, or being out in the community, I think health-care institutions can make a big difference in how the public perceives medicine. When we are out in their communities before the emergency strikes, we can build relationships and trust that is still lacking today. When we speak to their needs, acknowledging their concerns about vaccines and past medical exploitation, we show that we are not hiding anything from them and that we are ready to have an honest conversation. I believe that educating the public on vaccines, healthier lifestyles, addressing social determinants of health, and ensuring everyone has access to basic health care and how to access care will go a long way to reducing inequities. But hospitals, pharmaceutical companies, and governments must do the grassroots work of getting out into the communities, meeting people where they are, and listening to their concerns.

It took a miracle to bring together all our major institutions—government, health care, law enforcement, education, private industry, and more—to battle COVID-19, a ferocious unknown enemy. By all accounts, we seem to have won the war. What if we applied just some of that combined power of possibilities to other problems in our society?

ACKNOWLEDGMENTS

Writing this memoir has been a deeply personal and transformative experience, one that would not have been possible without the support and assistance of numerous individuals and organizations like Northwell Health. Michael Dowling, thank you for your authenticity and leadership and for demonstrating to the Northwell family and the world how to live a life of service, do good, embrace inclusivity, and address the important issues head-on simply because it's the right and just thing to do even if it is unpopular.

My heartfelt gratitude goes out to those who contributed to the creation of this book and helped shed light on important social injustice issues, inequities, the COVID-19 pandemic, and the significance of vaccines.

First, I would like to extend my deepest appreciation to the individuals who courageously shared their stories with me. Your openness and vulnerability have allowed me to delve into the complexities of social injustice, inequities, and the impact of the COVID-19 pandemic on marginalized communities. Your experiences serve as a powerful reminder of the urgent need for change and have inspired the narrative of this memoir.

I am indebted to the dedicated health-care professionals globally, and especially at Northwell Health, whom I have had the privilege of working with for thirty wonderful years, and the scientists who have worked tirelessly during the COVID-19 pandemic to protect and care for our communities. Your unwavering commitment to public health and the development of safe and effective vaccines has been instrumental in combating this global crisis. Your selflessness and expertise have saved countless lives. I am grateful for your contributions and to call you my colleagues.

My sincere appreciation goes to organizations and institutions that have championed the cause of social justice and equity. Your tireless efforts to address systemic inequalities and promote inclusivity have laid the foundation for a more just and compassionate society. Your advocacy and initiatives have provided the impetus for change and have been a driving force behind the themes explored in this memoir.

I have benefited greatly from the solid education provided by institutions in Jamaica and the United States that helped prepare me for success. Thanks to all the educators who believed in me even when I did not believe in myself. Through education, I have been afforded so many opportunities. I cannot thank my mentors, formal and informal, enough for sharing their most valuable resource—time—and their wisdom, which continues to impact my growth and development tremendously. Lynda Hartman and Maxine Cenac-Carrington, I will always treasure having you as mentors.

To the most important people in my life—my family and friends—thank you. To my parents, Basil and Hazel, and my grandparents, Norris and Harriet, thank you for teaching and demonstrating the values of respect, integrity, hard work, focus, determination, and service and for giving me a solid foundation to build on. Kadeem, my son, my first and forever love, you taught me from a young age what it means to unconditionally love and care about someone other than yourself. My brother, Garfield, my best friend, rock, and confidant, thank you for being my guiding light, a listening ear, a shoulder to cry on, and the one who will always tell me what is and not what I want to hear. Our many long talks under the mango tree as children growing up at Hartwell Gardens were not in vain. Many thanks to my other family members and friends for your unwavering support and encouragement throughout this journey. Your belief in me and willingness to listen and offer guidance have been invaluable. Your love and encouragement have sustained me during difficult times, and I am forever grateful.

My heartfelt thanks to my coauthor/editor, Joanne Skerrett, whose keen editorial eye and insightful feedback have helped shape this memoir into its final form. Your dedication to this project and commitment to amplifying important voices deserve special recognition.

Dr. Dave Livingstone, your keen eye for detail, insightful suggestions, and commitment to helping me shape my manuscript have truly elevated the quality of the book. Your feedback has been instrumental in refining my ideas and ensuring that the final product is polished and ready for publication.

I am deeply grateful to my book agent Sha-Shana Crichton for her unwavering belief in this project. After facing numerous rejections, her decision to champion this book and work tirelessly to bring it to fruition has been nothing short of remarkable. Her dedication, insight, and unwavering support have made all the difference, and I am profoundly thankful for her faith in both the book and in me. Without her willingness to take a chance, this project would not have seen the light of day. Thank you for making this dream a reality.

Thank you to the Northwell Marketing and Communications team for their unwavering commitment to amplifying the crucial message of vaccine advocacy and health equity. Their dedication and tireless efforts in pushing for exposure to tell my story have been instrumental in raising awareness and promoting positive change. Their passion for amplifying voices and advocating for public health has not gone unnoticed, and I am truly thankful for their invaluable support. Together, we are making a meaningful impact on our community and beyond. Thank you for your dedication to this vital cause.

Finally, I want to express my profound gratitude to the readers of this memoir. It is through your engagement and empathy that the stories within these pages find meaning and resonance. Your willingness to confront difficult subjects and engage in conversations about social justice and public health is crucial to fostering positive change. Thank you all for your support, guidance, and contributions. Together, we can strive for a more equitable and compassionate world.